# A Resilient Life:

## Learning to Thrive, not just survive, with rheumatoid arthritis

*Written by Kat Elton, OTR*

www.KatElton.com

**A Resilient Life: Learning to Thrive, not just survive with rheumatoid arthritis.**
By Kat Elton, OTR

Copyright © 2010 by Kat Elton
www.KatElton.com

Book Cover/ Interior design by Jarran Design

Library of Congress Control Number: 2009910569

Elton, Kat
A Resilient Life; Learning to Thrive, not just survive with rheumatoid arthritis/ Kat Elton.

ISBN **978-0-615-28923-6**

This book is strictly educational in nature and not to be used as specific health or medical advice. The information contained within this book is not intended or recommended to be used as treatment or diagnosis for any health problem. All matters concerning physical health should be supervised by a qualified health care practitioner knowledgeable in treating that particular condition. The author is not responsible for any unfavorable reactions to recommendations contained herein.

**The author has taken care to ensure the information in this book is accurate and up to date, however, as knowledge in medicine is constantly changing and new information discovered, changes in treatment occur. The reader is encouraged to acknowledge his/her unique situation when considering any recommendation in this book.**

**Ordering information:**
**To order copies of this book, please visit the following website:**
**www.katelton.com**

*To the Elton clan*
*And to all the amazing healers who, over the years,*
*have given me back my life*

# A Word About The Worksheets

At the end of each chapter you'll find worksheets. My suggestion is this; photocopy them and put them into a notebook. Fill them out as you read each chapter and, later, as things come up you can refer to your notebook. Together, with my guidance and your self- knowledge you will find that the answers you need are there.

Note: You may also download larger versions of the worksheets and have access to other resources online at **www.KatElton.com**.

# Table of Contents

# Table of Contents

# Introduction:
## A Resilient Life

Mae West once said, "Old age isn't for sissies," I say neither is arthritis. People with arthritis are some of the toughest people I know. Put a bunch of people with arthritis in a room with professional athletes and they'd have a lot to talk about: how to push through and go beyond a pain threshold that would stop most people in their tracks, how to ignore discomfort, how the snap, crackle, and popping joints between them could create a chorus, how to pick yourself up after a fall, what it's like to be alone out there. Professional athletes will brush off injuries because those injuries jeopardize their ability to participate in the next game. People with arthritis will brush off their pain because it jeopardizes their ability to participate, period.

When you are diagnosed with a chronic disease you soon confront one of the most humbling experiences of being human. In large part we are completely alone in our experience. The people around you can go on with their lives, yet you have to deal with this 24/7. Sometimes it may feel like you are treading water, other times that you are sinking and occasionally you get to swim. Your whole world has narrowed and widened at the same time. Narrowed, because you have this entity to constantly keep track of which can feel stifling. Widened, because you have been introduced to a whole new world-being a patient.

There is so much decision-making that you alone must make from what medications to take, how much to spend on things to ease your discomfort, and the limits you place on yourself and others so that you have enough energy to make it through the day. The internal dialogue can get very busy. Explaining it all to others may seem so difficult you don't even know where to begin. You alone end up juggling the busyness in your head. The fact is that having a chronic disease can isolate you from others both emotionally and physically. All of this is important to confront as early as possible in your process of living with chronic disease.

And then it's important to remember that for a penny to be a penny it has to have two sides. In life, for something to exist there must be an opposite to even it out. Night/day, love/hate, fear/trust, isolation/togetherness, and disease/ease. It is possible to thrive with rheumatoid arthritis as contradictory as this may seem at first. The road that leads there embraces both sides of the coin. The alone part can lead you toward taking responsibility, seeking out others to be on your healing team, which leads you to togetherness. You learn to live in both. You learn to see the opportunity that life has brought you; the opportunity to slow down, really look at yourself, and experience who you truly are.

Thriving with arthritis means you wake up every day and decide to thrive. In doing so you see that your greatest tool is your perspective, and attitude really is everything. You learn to be patient. You learn to transform your suffering into compassion, which literally means "to suffer with." You're humbled, time and time again, and then you're grateful. You work hard to do your homework but then you allow yourself to live in the unknown. At times all you can do is laugh at the absurdity of it all. Eventually you realize how truly resilient and strong you are.

There is richness in a life of thriving with chronic disease I doubt can be gained anywhere else. Through it all you must reach into the depths of your soul, be strong, savor the experience, and be grateful. It will transform you and I guarantee it will make you a better person. How you do this is up to you. The Golden Rule in this game is to keep trying, if you are doing that you are doing everything.

I didn't write this book because there is a lack of information about rheumatoid arthritis available. Actually, the amount of information we have today is mind-boggling. One trip to Barnes & Noble's, Amazon.com or Google will confirm this. I've been to them all, and guess what, I've found so many ways to beat this disease it's amazing any of us still have it!

How many of you would take 10,000 mg of vitamin C every day if it took away the pain? How many of you would stop eating wheat? Sleep on magnets? To those people who've cured their arthritis through any of these means I applaud you. The problem is, for 99.5% of us, it's not that simple and when we read about "Grandma's Arthritis Cures," or "The Cure For All Diseases," we are bound to get our hopes up.

I'm the type of person who can wear rose colored glasses. I'm grateful for this; they work for me most of the time. But they can also get me into trouble. Trouble, because time after time I've convinced myself that this will be it. I'll tell myself, "Of course, humans can't produce vitamin C and because I don't like orange juice I've let the arthritis run rampant in my body! BIG mistake." And then the rose colored glasses come off. Time after time, high hopes, hopes dashed, until I can't help but wonder, "Why me?"

At that point, I will inevitably hear from my Aunt Matilda, who has a friend with a son, whose cousin went to Mexico and came back in glowing health. "Well, shoot," I have to wonder, "Why is everyone coming up here from south of the border if they have the cure for one of the nemesis of our time?"

This is about the time I turn back to the doctors to learn more about the chronic, progressive, disabling illness that not only attacks my joints but also my eyes, skin, organs, and most horribly my sense of humor. To top it off it's all because my immune system is defective and has decided to attack my own tissues. So it's all my fault, just as I suspected, and I go back to the books.

According to the experts, in order to best manage this disabling disease I need to think positive, do  range of motion exercises every day, protect my joints, swim, watch what I eat, do visualization, get good sleep every night, take medications as prescribed, avoid stress... wait a second, do I get to live a life here? And then the realization hits me that this is my life, this is my chance to create a life that I can be proud of.

The reason I'm writing this book for you is precisely because you don't need to be told what to do.  As someone who has spent every moment since age two with arthritis and has worked as an occupational therapist I consider myself more than a little qualified. But for these reasons I know wholeheartedly that when it comes to rheumatoid arthritis and chronic disease in general there are no absolutes.

When I was young I learned very quickly that when an adult said "This won't hurt" they were lying. So I decided that before anyone did anything to me they had to explain what they were going to do in detail. I remember going to the dentist to get a bunch of teeth pulled and being forewarned that I would bleed a lot because of the aspirin I was taking for the arthritis. Just that little bit of information allowed me to prepare myself for what was to come and helped me to feel like I was part of the process. I never lost the need to feel that way. When you have rheumatoid arthritis there are many times when things happen to you and you can easily feel as if your life is spiraling out of your control. I've always felt strongly that knowledge is power and that you never run out of options. These two ideas have kept me going when the going got tough.

My goal is to have this book give you the knowledge and the options you will need to live well with rheumatoid arthritis. Each chapter addresses a different issue or area of concern that I've encountered numerous times throughout my life. Inside each chapter you will find personal experiences, knowledge I've gained, and tools to use. Use this book like a toolbox. Use the tools when you need them and when you don't be assured that they are there. The best tools won't be the one's I'll give you though; they will be the ones you discover within yourself.

Being a patient has always been a part of my life and as a kid my parents always made the experience a special one. I'd get dressed up, drive across the George Washington Bridge to Columbia Presbyterian Hospital which was an exciting experience. After all I was going to New York City! My Mom and I would arrive at Dr. Jacob's office where I'd feel very grown up reading magazines while I waited to see the doctor. Okay, they were Highlight magazines for kids but I still felt very mature reading them. Once I was in the office Dr. Jacobs would examine my joints and talk to my Mom about how I was doing. When I was in Dr. Jacob's office I was the center of attention. My needs were being addressed and I felt cared for. Even getting my blood taken wasn't so bad. I'd feel very brave by not making a fuss when they poked me with the needle and I still remember the stuffed animals and pictures on the wall to take my mind off the pain.

Looking back with what I know now about healing, Columbia Presbyterian, and Dr. Jacobs, did everything right. Being a patient there did not go hand in hand with fear, apprehension, anxiety, or frustration but instead gave me the experience of feeling good.

I wish I could say it was always that way but given my long history as a patient it was inevitable that at some point I'd eventually experience less compassionate care. The first and probably most dramatic example of this happened before my *first hand surgery. Weeks earlier I had learned that I had ruptured one of the tendons that lifted my ring finger and I knew I was in deep trouble.*

*I was in the office of one of the top hand surgeons in the country and was being examined by a Fellow, a young doctor who was receiving training to specialize in hand surgery. This young doctor had swooped into the room, grabbed my painful hand, and started measuring my range of motion, blissfully unaware of my winces as he pushed and pulled on my joints. Abruptly, he looked down at my arm and dropped it. "What is that!" he said, and I looked down. I had suddenly started breaking out in angry red welts. "Looks like hives to me," I said. At the time I was not very aware of my emotional reactions and I still thought stoicism was the best way to approach my situation. However, it was apparent to me that anxious response to this guy's utter disrespect and disregard were causing me to break out in hives.*

*He left the room and I tried to calm my body. Minutes later he came back with my x-rays. He took one look at them and exclaimed in an excited voice, "Wow, look at this, I've never seen anything like it, not even in a textbook!" and then ran out of the room to fetch the other Fellows. Here I was, breaking out in hives because one of my worst fears, surgery, was coming to fruition and I had five doctors crammed into my tiny exam room "oohing" and "ahhing" at the horrible state of my wrist joint.*

*All I can say now is that it's a good thing this guy had decided to be a surgeon. Ninety percent of the time his rudeness would be irrelevant because his patients would be unconscious. And luckily for me, my hand surgeon, Dr. Melone, turned out to be a star. To this day he is one of my heroes.*

*I've learned a lot throughout my years as a patient, and also as an occupational therapist who has been on the other side of the exam table. And I've decided that for me, if a healthcare provider wants to keep me as a patient they have to meet a high standard. I've decided this because, in varying degrees, they have my life in their hands. And my precious life is not to be taken lightly.*

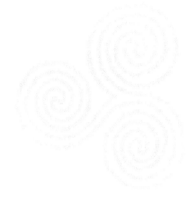

# Chapter One:
## The Art and Science of Being a Patient

*"The good physician treats the disease; the great physician treats the person who has the disease."*
*-- Sir William Osler*

Once you are diagnosed with a chronic disease you automatically assume another role in life, that of a patient. This role requires a lot of knowledge, fortitude, and diligence. There are many reasons for this not the least of which is that you come into it in a vulnerable state. You don't become a patient when you are in top form; there are no parties to symbolize it. Think about roles that you've assumed throughout your life, daughter/son, graduate, worker, mother/father, husband/wife. All of which come with new roles and responsibilities, but also with fanfare and celebration. You can say to the world, "I am a teacher," "I am so-and-so's wife," and the response is inevitably positive. Imagine saying, "I am a patient now." Not the same, I'm guessing. Yet, as a patient there is a lot to do: find a doctor, learn to negotiate the insurance system, keep track of medications and side effects, manage symptoms, manage the money it takes, adjust to this new identity, and find the time and energy for it all. You might as well have a new job.

Being a patient is a very humbling experience, it doesn't matter if you are a CEO of a company or work in a factory. Once you become a patient it will seem that your time is no longer valuable, your modesty will be checked at the door, and you are almost guaranteed to encounter at least one health care professional who lacks an empathy chip. You may experience gross insensitivity, arrogance, misplaced humor, and disrespect. All in the space of fifteen minutes or less and usually after a forty five minute wait.

There is no prerequisite for health practitioners to have a high emotional quotient, it's their IQ that's accounted for. If you are diligent you will find one with both and yet you can't back out unless you get better. Unfortunately, with a chronic disease remission is possible, but patient hood will most likely be a part of your life for the rest of your life. Do I sound like the glass is half empty? Do you want to kick something now? Good, because that will spur you to action. Being a patient is serious and can be life-threatening. I'm not talking about the disease, it's being in the system that can kill you.

Here are the facts. According to the Journal of American Medical Association medical care is the third leading cause of death in this country. Imagine a huge plane going down every day of the year and killing all its passengers and you'd be coming close. Here are some statistics:

- 106,000 negative effects from properly prescribed pharmaceutical drugs
- 80,000 infections in hospitals
- 20,000 other errors in hospitals
- 12,000 unnecessary surgeries
- 7,000 medication errors in hospitals
- Total of medically induced deaths, 225,000

This doesn't even include events that don't result in death. According to the Institute of Medicine in a report brief in July 2006, "There are at least 1.5 million preventable adverse drug events that occur in the United States every year. The true number may be much higher." The report also stated that a hospital patient can expect on average to be subjected to more than one medication error every day. As a result once you enter the system you are playing Russian roulette. This is precisely why it is imperative to not only know what you're getting into, but to learn quickly to take the reins and be an active, educated consumer.

## The Challenges of Being a Patient

The first and most important piece of this is to find a doctor you respect, trust, and just downright like. The vast majority of patients end up with doctors who don't fit this description and stay with them because they don't know of other options or are afraid to be labeled as a doctor shopper. Learn to shop, I say! It may be difficult at first, but in the long run you'll be eternally grateful to yourself that you did.

In the book "Blink" by Malcolm Gladwell, he describes an interesting study by a medical researcher named Wendy Levinson. She recorded hundreds of conversations between doctors and patients, half of whom had been sued at least twice. She found a curious difference between the doctors who'd been sued and those that hadn't. The doctors who hadn't been sued spent more than three minutes longer with each patient, said more orienting comments such as, "I will leave time for your questions," engaged in active listening and were more likely to laugh and be funny. There was no difference in the amount or quality of medical information they gave their patients.

In another study the tone of the doctor was analyzed for qualities like warmth, dominance, hostility, and anxiousness. The study found that doctors who were sued sounded dominant. Skill level, experience and training had nothing to do with it. So what does this tell you? It tells me that someone who sues is angry and feels harmed. It also tells me that words and disrespect can harm just as much, if not more, than physical damage.

The doctor-patient relationship can be strained in other ways. On average, doctors interrupt their patients after 23 seconds due to their concerns about limited time. However, if the doctor doesn't interrupt, on average a patient will only talk for 90 seconds. The important point to this is that most often people won't verbalize their most worrisome complaint until the end of the visit.

I can relate to this. Deep down, you hope and pray that if you don't mention the complaint it will go away on its own. Mentioning it makes it real. In the best of circumstances sitting in a doctor's office is an anxiety producing event, otherwise the term "white coat effect" would not exist. Then you add the depersonalization and embarrassment of the process and all of a sudden you are a number, a statistic, part of a group you'd never asked to join. And you're embarrassed by all the fuss. You are robbing time from your loved ones. You are in the spotlight, but not in a good way.

Dr. Barry Bob, a physician for 30 years, wrote an amazing book called *"Communication Skills That Heal, a Practical Approach to a New Professionalism in Medicine."* It is a book that is written for doctors but has a lot to tell patients. He makes a few very insightful points in his book. He states that a patient's biggest wish is to have their isolation relieved. He says that listening well involves being listened to and the ability to hear with focused attention. He says that shame and anxiety interfere with hearing. He says that due to decreased reimbursement rates physicians are feeling multiple pressures from hospitals and insurance companies to see more patients in less time and are themselves victimized by the trend towards treating pathologies instead of people. Doctors are working longer hours and are having less free time. Huge malpractice costs are causing some to retire early. The predominant feeling is that there is no time to listen to a person's life story, effective treatment doesn't require it. He correctly states that "Patients come to the medical establishment for treatment and to the alternative community for healing. This creates a split or division of care that is inherently unhealthy and denies both patients and practitioners to symbiotic benefits that are possible." He insightfully brings home the point that doctors, and all health professionals for that matter, are people too.

So, when you are with your doctor notice how you feel, how he or she treats you. Do you feel listened to? Do you feel as if you have enough time to ask questions? Do you feel respected? Does your doctor know who you are? Are you feeling so anxious much of the time that you aren't hearing what your doctor tells you? If you respect your doctor's abilities but are unsure of some of these answers, it may behoove you to give him or her the benefit of the doubt and look at your behavior. Are you telling your doctor that you have questions at the beginning of the visit or do you wait until the end to squeeze them in? Are you offering helpful feedback to your doctor?

Remember, your relationship with your doctor is one of the most important relationships you are ever going to have in your life so it is vital to examine it and work hard to make it as productive as possible. It is important to be proactive instead of reactive.

Assume that you found a doctor whose abilities and knowledge you respect and trust. That is all you need to create a positive, and dare I say, a healing relationship even given the pressures of modern medicine. Let us see how to begin.

## *Doctors are People Too*

It takes two to tango in any relationship. The one difficulty with the doctor- patient relationship that is apparent from the start is the inequity of power. To state it one way, your doctor literally holds your life in his or her hands. Your doctor will prescribe drugs and other treatments that have the potential to give you your life back. The passivity that is encouraged during the process of being a patient further influences this inequality of power. Think back to a time when you went to the doctor with someone, say a family member other than a child, and how they behaved once they donned the infamous "one-size fits nobody" gown. Now think about your behavior in this circumstance. How do you change, if at all? You may notice subtle changes like increased passivity, tentativeness, or vulnerability. Part of the psychology of this is where the medical system has placed doctors, on the top. Part of this is that when you are facing a serious illness you need comfort, reassurance, and safety. Innately we look to a parental figure for this.

And partly it is the overwhelming amount of choices we face as a patient. In a book by Barry Schwartz, called *The Paradox of Choice* he talks about how although having some choice is positive too many choices can paralyze people and make their ultimate decision less satisfying. He mentions a study that found 65% of healthy people said that if they got cancer they would prefer to choose their treatment, of people with cancer, 88% said that they would prefer not to choose their treatment. The amount of choices we face as a patient are numerous and ongoing, something I'll discuss more later. Letting someone tell us what to do will take away a number of the choices we have to make on a daily basis and when facing a chronic illness this can be a huge relief.

Now, let us stare these issues in the face. The inherit inequality of power in the doctor's office, the innate need for comfort and reassurance, the paradox of choice, the vulnerable state that is a given when you are seeing a doctor, and a passivity that is encouraged by the system. Can we create a healing relationship in the midst of all this? Yes, we can, and I'll tell you why. Doctors are people too. And if he or she is worth his stuff, he wants this as much as you do.

Pretend you are your doctor. What kind of patient would you prefer to see in your office, one that is passive, tentative, letting you call all the shots ,or one that is prepared, respectful and is able to articulate his or her needs, expectations and hopes? I'm guessing the latter. When I was in college I was fortunate enough to find a doctor who encouraged me to talk about how I was feeling. I'll never forget having Dr. Bluestone tell me "Fine is not an answer" when he asked me how I was doing and I inevitably gave that one word reply. It took me aback at first because I wasn't used to having a doctor who wanted to listen to how I really felt. Up until then, fine worked, well, just fine. But Dr. Bluestone's response encouraged me to really think about how I was doing and empowered me to get into the driver's seat when it came to monitoring my arthritis symptoms. Ultimately, doctors benefit from engaged patients who communicate with them. Patients want engaged doctors who communicate with them. Sounds like a win-win situation to me.

## *Become a Person, Not a Patient*

Let's take apart this inherit inequality of power. How does one even the score? This is achieved by becoming a person, not a patient. First, let's talk body language. When I visit the doctor, I always have a serious discussion with him when I'm at his level not when I am on the table on my back.  Preferably, I am dressed. I always bring something to read when I go to the doctor so if I have a long wait I don't get frustrated. I psych myself up for the visit by reminding myself that I am the one in charge, it's my body after all. If I decide to take the doctors' recommendations at face value and follow them it's my choice but I don't have to do this if I don't want to. I'm in the driver's seat.  Ultimately, my doctor is a consultant, albeit a very educated, and informed one, and I use him as such.

Before I visit the doctor I really think about what I want from the visit, what are my goals, and I write these down. Then I write down questions that reflect these goals. When the visit begins I clearly state what my goals are. Then, when I am asking my questions I start with the most important one first so we don't run out of time. If it is the one that concerns me most I tell my doctor this and if I don't get time for all of my questions I ask my doctor if I can leave them with him to respond to at his earliest convenience. Speaking for myself, my ultimate goal is always remission and I tell my doctor this. "I'm working to achieve remission and I'd like your help in doing this." It feels so good to say it and brings you respect.

I keep it lighthearted whenever possible and get to know my doctor and his staff. When I ask, "How are you?," I mean it. When the nurse comes to check my vital signs, I always ask her about herself and I remember to follow up during the next visit. If I like my doctor's tie I say, so. I ask how his vacation was, and I really listen to his answer. By creating a light yet caring conversation with the staff and really listening to their answers you are setting the tone for the rest of the visit. Remember what Dr. Barry Bob said, "Listening well involves being listened to and the ability to hear with focused attention." If you begin by listening to the doctor or nurse they will be more apt to listen back and starting a visit on a person to person note creates an actual real relationship that is an excellent basis for compassionate care. Ninety nine percent of health care professionals do what they do because they genuinely want to help people and it's important to remember this.

I also come in with the attitude that I will be accomplishing something positive during my time there. Emotions are contagious. Even if physically I'm doing worse I'm still on the road to remission, I just haven't put all the pieces of the puzzle together yet. If I come in with this attitude my doctor will feel this and automatically be more likely to be positive with me. I don't suppress my negative emotions with my doctor but he also knows that I'm not there for psychotherapy. Telling him I'm angry at my body is useful information but I don't need him to stop everything and say ,"Tell me how you feel about this." I'll leave that to another practitioner to address if I so choose. This respects his time limits, but gets your needs met. I also utilize the nursing staff. When I call a doctor I always ask to have the doctor or his nurse get back to me because this will inevitably get me a quicker response. If I need to speak with the doctor I ask when he does call backs and I make myself available at that time so I don't have to sit around the rest of the day twiddling my thumbs.

These actions take me out of the role of the stereotypical patient and into the role of a proactive person who is working within the limitations of my doctor's time to get my needs met. They put me in the driver's seat and even out the inequity of power that is inherent in the system.

So what about the need for reassurance and vulnerability that comes with being a patient? This is where trusted friends and family can be a huge help. If you can have someone with you during a visit to the doctor they can ask questions you may not think of when you're under stress. He/she can also help you to remember answers to questions and advocate for you when you are feeling vulnerable. If you can't, or prefer not to have someone with you during an appointment, you can consult with them following a visit to go over what was said and done. They may think of something you forgot to ask or remember a concern you had a month ago that is no longer on your mind. A trusted adviser can also help with the paradox of choice when you are having difficulty making a decision about what to do.

With the immense number of choices patients face these days it is important to think about what works for you. Do you like to learn as much as you can about every option available or do you prefer to trust the advice of your doctor? Personally, I'm in the former category. Before embarking on any new medicine regime or treatment I'll be busy on the internet reading and talking to people about what I've learned. When I was younger I was in the latter category and at the time that worked for me as well. The point is, know yourself and feel good about it. Feeling good about your choices may be the most important step of all. All of these actions are positive, proactive, and put you in the driver's seat working towards creating a positive relationship with your doctor.

## *Other Health Care Providers*

Now let's talk about other kinds of healthcare practitioners and why they are important. As an occupational therapist I'm a bit biased, I admit, but I think absolutely everyone diagnosed with rheumatoid arthritis should see an occupational therapist within six months of treatment. It has always been a pet peeve of mine that I inevitably start working with someone after they've had surgery. Only then am I able to educate my clients about things that may have prevented the need for surgery in the first place or at least improved their quality of life beforehand. Occupational therapists can help in a myriad of ways, but their specialty is function. OT's help you to improve your quality of life and ability to function at your optimal level through education, compensatory techniques, adaptive equipment, and exercise.

Physical therapists are also extremely useful in providing an exercise program designed to keep you strong while maintaining the integrity of your joints. Your doctor may or may not bring up the subject of therapy but you can always request a prescription for yourself. I've done this a lot and never had a doctor turn me down. And once again, do your homework. It is important to find the right fit with your therapist and especially important to work with someone who knows about the specific issues that people with rheumatoid arthritis face. You can do this by asking for recommendations from your doctor, nurse, friends, or by calling the Arthritis Foundation. Then speak to the therapist prior to your appointment and ask them questions about how much they've worked with people with arthritis. As a good friend of mine who has had arthritis since childhood and also happens to be a physical therapist pointed out, you're not looking for someone who works with the local basketball team but you're also not looking for someone who primarily works with eighty year olds who have osteoporosis. You are looking for a happy medium, someone whose abilities you have confidence in and you like and trust.

There are other health professionals who can be of great benefit but may be harder to find. These include health psychologists who specialize in chronic issues and chronic pain specialists.

To wrap up, let me summarize specific red flags to watch out for when choosing a health care practitioner as well as signs that you have found a good fit.

## Red flags:

- You feel that questions are not welcome.

- You feel rushed during your visit.

- He/she is not forthcoming and you are constantly feeling uninformed with regard to your care.

- He/she is condescending, cold, abrupt, or patronizing.

- There is a lack of continuity in your care. For example if you feel that you constantly have to repeat your history to your doctor and he/she is not remembering you from one visit to the next.

- You continually have extremely long waits to see the doctor. This may mean that he/she is disorganized with other aspects of handling their office.

## Gold Stars:

- You feel comfortable asking your questions and are open and honest with your doctor about your concerns.

- You receive call backs in a timely manner.

- You feel respected and listened to.

- Your doctor has a sense of humor.

- Your doctor remembers things that you have told him in previous visits.

- Your doctor is willing and able to discuss long-term goals and the possibility of remission.

- Your doctor has helpful and friendly office staff. This most likely means that they are happy in their jobs and will take pride in their work.

## And finally, a wrap up of how to be an assertive, proactive patient:

- Come into the doctor's office prepared with your questions and state the most important and/or disconcerting one first.

- Write down answers to your questions immediately after or during the visit.

- If you feel more comfortable bring a trusted friend or family member with you to the visit. Be clear with them prior to the visit about your goals, questions, and concerns so that they will know what to listen for and ask about during the visit.

- Without faking it, come into each visit with your doctor with an upbeat attitude, knowing that you will be accomplishing something positive during your time there. Get to know the office staff and nursing staff so that they will remember you from visit to visit.

- Let your body language reflect an assertive attitude by utilizing eye contact and staying at your doctor's level whenever possible.

- Come prepared for each visit by writing down relevant symptoms and concerns for your doctor so that you can discuss them with him in a thoughtful, concise, and specific manner. Remember that he's not a mind reader; he won't be able to help you unless he knows what's going on.

## *Managing Medications*

Rheumatoid arthritis and medications are like peanut butter and jelly; whether you like the combination or not the two will go together at some point in time. It's too bad that it's not as simple as making a sandwich because with medications there are side effects. Medications are potent substances and by definition any drug will be toxic at a high enough level. Combined with the statistic regarding medication errors I stated earlier (1.5 million preventable adverse drug events yearly), it is important to be diligent with understanding and monitoring how your medications are affecting you, both good and bad. The first step in this is in the doctor's office before you decide to embark on a new drug regime.

### The questions to ask and get acceptable answers to include:

- Do you have any written material or a web site to look up about this medication?
- How should I take the medication?
- What are common side effects and other changes to watch out for?
- How long before it starts to work?
- How will it interact with any other medications I'm taking?
- Are there foods or supplements to avoid while I'm taking this medication?
- How long will I need it?

The last question is especially important because some drugs are bridge drugs, which means they are meant to be taken to relieve your symptoms until another long term drug starts to work in your system. You should be informed and agree on exactly what is being done during each step of your care, knowing how long each treatment will last and how you should feel during the process, as well as understanding and being on board with the long term plan for your medical treatment.

Once you have decided to start taking a drug there are ways to avoid errors in dispensing and administering it.

## Here are some ideas:

- Establish yourself with a pharmacy that you trust. The first time you fill a prescription ask to have the pharmacist explain side effects and what is written on the label to you. This assures that they have filled the right medication and the instructions for taking the drug jive with what your doctor told you.

- Obtain printed information from your pharmacist each time you fill a prescription to have on hand if any unusual changes do occur.

- Make sure your pharmacy keeps a list of all your medications in their computer. Once again this safeguards taking two drugs that interact negatively with each other. There is an excellent web site on Medscape that can be found by typing in *www.medscape.com/druginfo/druginterchecker*. At this web site you can type in all of the medications you are taking and it will check to see if there are any harmful interactions between them.

- Read the label every time you take a medication to confirm that you're taking the right one and keep your medications away from other prescriptions that other members of your household may be taking.

- Never store them in direct light, heat, or humidity.

- Never take anyone else's prescription or one that has expired.

- Dispose of old, expired drugs in a safe, environmentally friendly way. This can be done by locating a drug recycling program in your area or household hazardous waste facilities. Never flush old medications down the toilet or put them in the sink. Sewage treatment plants are not designed to treat all substances contained in medications and they end up in rivers, creeks and our drinking water. A US geological survey found evidence of antibiotics, birth control pills, and other drugs in our surface waters, so if we're not careful we may be inadvertently drinking each other's medications and feeding them to our fish and other wild creatures.

- Learn about any adverse drug/supplement combinations. One good reference book is titled *A-Z Guide to Drug-Herb-Vitamin Interactions, How to Improve Your Health and Avoid Problems When Using Common Medications*, written by Schuyler W. Lininger Jr.

Know that unusual side effects do occur and it's NOT in your head. Don't be afraid to call and talk to your doctor if any unusual changes do occur when you are taking a new drug. Just because something has worked for a while or in the past doesn't mean this will always be the case. Your personal physiology and tolerance level are always in flux. It's always better to be cautious, in the end you will be happy you were because you'll be able to reassure yourself and have one less thing to worry about.

The final very important thing to keep in mind is that you need to be careful with consulting doctors who aren't specialists in rheumatology. When you see a general practitioner or any other medical doctor for a non arthritis related issue and they prescribe medication it is always smart to call your rheumatologist and let them know. You have an immune system that likes to go into overdrive and the last thing you want is to inadvertently be revving it up.

## Straight Talk about Surgery

Surgery is never fun, but the results can be. It's always fun to be in less pain and have more function. When you have rheumatoid arthritis for long enough the surgery issue is bound to come up eventually so the more you know beforehand the better off you'll be when the time comes. I'm not going to discuss specifics, as techniques are always improving and options change, but I will help you to understand how surgery can help.

There are two reasons why surgery should be considered for people with RA; to decrease pain and to increase function. Sometimes the decision is a no-brainer as it was for me when I had my right wrist fused. In my case, the right wrist was the first place I got arthritis so by the time I was 23 the wrist had already been through 20 years of siege.

I was in occupational therapy school at the time, ironically enough, studying hand therapy, when a tendon popped in my right hand. That night, studying biomechanics of the hand, I realized my ring finger didn't want to lift up, which disturbed me to say the least. The next day I told my instructor, who was also my O.T., and she immediately sent me to a hand surgeon. As it turns out one of the long bones in my arm, the ulna, had moved which ended up shredding my tendons until finally one of them popped. As it also turns out I had only one wrist bone left, the lunate, and it was hanging out off in space somewhere doing absolutely no good. One look at this situation and it was an easy decision to fuse the joint entirely. I've never looked back.

The only sad thing about the whole situation, besides the fact that I had to have arthritis at all, is that my occupational therapist had mentioned to me months prior that it might be good to have my hand looked at by a surgeon. When I mentioned this to my rheumatologist at the time he blew up and yelled that she had no right to suggest such a thing, that was his job and the subject was dropped. He got to be top dog again, and I ended up with three tendons that will never be the same. Doesn't sound like much of a fair deal to me. Needless to say, I've learned the hard way how imperative it is to find a good doctor.

Back to improved function and deceased pain. My wrist fusion accomplished both. My wrist was fused, which took away a painful joint, and improved stability which increased function. My shredded extensor tendons were reattached, giving me back the ability to use those fingers. As I said, a no-brainer.

Before my surgery I asked my hand surgeon, Dr Melone, if he could fix my pinky which had had something called a boutonniere deformity. What that means is that the middle finger joint, called the inter-phalangeal joint, was fixed in a bent position. This was caused by years of being stretched over an inflamed joint and then falling to the side which changed the angle of pull there. My surgeon looked at my pinky, looked at me, and asked, "Does it hurt?" "Well, no."Are you able to use it? "Well, yes." The real reason I wanted him to fix it was because I was embarrassed to have a funny looking finger, not on the list of appropriate reasons to have surgery.

So, anytime a health care practitioner brings up the subject of surgery remember those two words, pain and function. If the surgery isn't improving one, or preferably both of these things, just say no. If it is, it's time to start doing your homework.

### Here are some questions to ponder:

- What are the risks of having the surgery?

- What are the surgical options for me?

- What could happen if I don't have it?

- Are there other ways to accomplish the same goals of the surgery? (i.e. splinting or bracing)

### If, after considering these questions you decide to have surgery done, consider these questions:

- What should I expect the recovery time to be?
- How should I expect to feel during recovery?
- How long before I can return to work?
- How long will I be in the hospital?
- Will I need physical or occupational therapy after the surgery?
- Who will be available to help me out during my recovery time?
- Last but not least, how much will my insurance pay for?

The final piece of this puzzle is to find the best surgeon for the job. With a surgeon you will be less concerned about developing a healing relationship and more concerned about how experienced he or she is with this particular surgery, who is on their surgical team, and the hospital they practice out of. The hospital is important because it is during post surgical care that medical mistakes would most likely occur. Finding a surgeon won't be too difficult, your rheumatologist should be able to provide you with some names, but asking friends and family is smart too. Word of mouth is a powerful tool.

**Now, you've found your surgeon and are ready to prepare for an overnight hospitalization.**

**Time for another list:**
- Ask who will be in charge of your care during your hospitalization.

- Try to arrange someone to be with you as much as possible. This person will act as an advocate, as you won't be able to advocate for yourself for much of the time, and will be an extra hand to help you when you need it.

- Pack an overnight bag and include comfortable clothes and toiletries that will make you feel good. Believe me, having a lotion or soap with a comforting smell will do wonders for improving how you feel, and soft PJ's to put on will lift your spirits.

Once you are in the hospital pay attention to the care you are receiving. Use the person who is with you to help ensure that you are getting the correct medications by having them double check with the nurse anytime they give you something. If you have any allergies make sure that the entire staff knows this. A list of your allergies may be placed in red on the front of your chart so that everyone can see them, or on your medical bracelet. If the hospital has another policy for this make sure you know what it is and that they are following it. Get to know the names of all your caregivers and make sure they confirm your identity before giving you any treatment. Don't hesitate to remind people to wash their hands before touching you and this includes any visitors you may have. Speaking of visitors, although it is important to have someone with you, too many visitors can zap your energy really fast, and your energy needs to go towards healing your body. Allow family and close friends only and even limit phone calls, there will be plenty of time for well wishes later. Surgery is an intense experience and the decision to have it should not be taken lightly, but the benefits that can be gained should not be taken lightly either. Improved function and decreased pain can do much for your quality of life.

Hopefully by now you've realized that you are the most important member of your health care team. You and only you are in charge of your body. Anyone else is a consultant who will provide you with information and resources to make decisions you can feel good about. You know your body better than anyone on the planet which means that you can trust yourself to know when things are awry. You have the right to be respected. You have the right to find healthcare practioners that you respect. You have the ability to create a positive, productive relationship with your healthcare providers. As RA is constantly in flux, your needs will be in flux and you have a duty to yourself to address those needs as they come up. Becoming a proactive patient is empowering, will definitely improve your life, and can literally save your life. You owe it to yourself to make the effort.

# *Chapter One Worksheet*

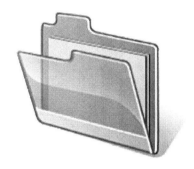

- Doctor Visit Checklist

# DOCTOR VISIT CHECKLIST

Date: _____ Appointment with: _____

My goals for this visit: _____

_____

_____

My long term goals: _____

_____

_____

Symptoms I've been having since my last visit: _____

_____

_____

Medications I am taking:                          Supplements/ Vitamins I am taking:

_____          _____

_____          _____

_____          _____

_____          _____

_____          _____

_____          _____

_____          _____

_____          _____

_____          _____

_____          _____

_____          _____

_____          _____

_____          _____

_____          _____

_____          _____

_____          _____

_____          _____

_____          _____

Specific questions I have about my treatment: (Write answers underneath)

1. _____

_____

_____

2. _____

_____

_____

3. _____

_____

_____

4. _____

_____

_____

5. _____

_____

_____

6. _____

_____

_____

Other information from my doctor I need to remember:_____

_____

_____

_____

_____

_____

_____

_____

_____

_____

_____

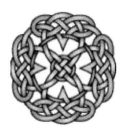

*I'm in the unique position of never being aware of life without pain. I've often wondered which is worse, having such a long history with pain as my constant companion, or knowing what it's like to be pain free and then having it taken away. The interesting thing is that I never consider myself to have chronic pain. I've always thought of chronic pain sufferers as being in a distinct category of people that are separate from me and I've realized that this is because my pain is so changeable. Ask me one minute and my thumb might be on the radar, five minutes later it's my ankle. It comes and goes, surges and recedes, gets stuck and throbbing. It can be sharp, sludgy, hot, and transient. It can radiate off every cell in my body. It is so changeable I think it definitely has a mind of its own. It's not chronic, it is a series of acute issues that constantly keep me guessing.*

*The other day I mentioned to a very good friend that I had gone on a bike ride. It somehow came up that it hurt. My friend Mark was surprised that bike riding caused me pain. He said, "I thought you were doing better, didn't you also do a two hour hike over the weekend?" It struck me, yet again, that regardless of how well I know them the majority of people are clueless about the level of pain I live with. My pain isn't something I broadcast because from a very young age I came to think that since there was nothing anyone could do anyway it was a waste of breath to bring it up. When I did mention my arthritis I would inevitably hear one of two things. "You're too young!" to which I replied "I agree!" or "I have arthritis too, sometimes when it rains I can feel it," to which I remained silent. These days I'll mention the state of pain only if someone else asks or if it is going to impinge upon my ability to do something with them. No need to go into the long list otherwise. And no need to mention that when I think hard I can remember times I haven't been in pain.*

*My pain was actually never addressed with me in a clinical setting until very recently. The first time that a doctor asked if I wanted to take a pain medicine I just stared at her blankly thinking, "Aren't I just supposed to suck it up?" This is because when I was young very little was really known about pain. The prevailing thought was that narcotics, the only available options for pain back then, were addictive and needed to be avoided like the plague.*

*So grinning and bearing it was the status quo. And when pain's all you know and the people who surround you have no language for it, there's literally nothing to talk about. I speak Russian and you speak Chinese so we just end up smiling and nodding at each other. This was long before federal law created the inevitable question you now get at the doctor's office of "Rate your pain on a scale of one to ten." During that time many physicians still believed babies didn't feel pain.*

*I spent the majority of my life in this invisible world that for me was starkly real but for others was based on belief. My pain was only recognized if another went out of their way to do so. And because there was no dialog I was never fully aware of the scale of the pain that I dealt with. Throughout my young life I did have a few reality checks though, times that I suffered an acute injury that for many people would have them on their backs screaming, and for me was just another bad pain day.*

*One time I specifically remember was in the fifth grade. My family was on the first day of a weeklong ski vacation. We were at Hunter Mountain in New York State and would be heading north to Vermont after the day of skiing. I was skiing down the hill and realized my boots were too loose. Since I couldn't tighten them myself I skied faster to catch up to my Dad.*

*Unfortunately, I hit a bump and fell, lodging my right foot half in and half out of the boot. It hurt a lot. The ski patrol came and asked me to stand on my foot and I told them I couldn't. They didn't seem to believe me and kept asking and I kept insisting. Finally, they took me down to the first aid station in one of their sleds. At the first aid station they again asked me to stand on my foot. Yet again I said I couldn't. After a few more rounds of this they let me leave and my family and I drove north to Vermont to continue our vacation. I didn't sleep or eat much that night and hopped around the cabin we were staying at whenever I needed to move. My foot throbbed and I still couldn't stand on it. The next morning it still wasn't better so my parents took me to the urgent care center in town. Luckily they took me right to x-ray where they discovered I had a broken leg. I had a broken leg for almost twenty-four hours before anyone discovered it and I was only ten.*

*Years later I thought about this incident and realized that I wasn't responding to the severe pain I must have had in the way most kids would have which is why it took so long for anyone to figure out what was wrong. I also thought about how I responded to the disbelief that I couldn't stand on my foot. I didn't get angry, instead I became resigned. I was* resigned to the fact of the disbelief and steadfast in protecting myself from further harm by not standing on my broken leg. The fact is that disbelief was something I encountered all the time which was another reason not to engage in a conversation around pain. Pain is a uniquely personal experience, easier to disbelieve than to understand.

 Consider this quote from the book by Elaine Scarry, The Body in Pain, "When one speaks about "one's own physical pain" and about "another person's pain, one might almost appear to be speaking about two wholly distinct orders of events. For the person who's pain it is, it is "effortlessly" grasped (that is, even with the most heroic effort it cannot not be grasped) while for the person outside the sufferers body, what is "effortless" is not grasping it (it is easy to remain wholly unaware of its existence; even with effort one may remain in doubt about its existence or retain the astonishing freedom of denying its existence, and, finally, if with the best effort of sustained attention one successfully apprehends it, the aversiveness of the "it" one apprehends will only be a shadowy fraction of the actual "it") Thus pain comes unsharably into our midst as at once that which cannot be denied and that which cannot be confirmed." " ....to have great pain is to have certainty; to hear that another person has pain is to have doubt. (The doubt of other persons, here as elsewhere, amplifies the suffering of those already in pain.)"

I've lived this reality for so long that I experienced what seems like every kind of disbelief possible. I spent a summer repeatedly being stopped in my tracks and doubling over in pain while encountering disbelief that my stomach hurt that much until an ulcer was finally discovered. I came across disbelief in the neighborhood kids who wanted me to keep on *playing long after my body was crying out for rest. Summer camp counselors, doctors, parents, ski patrol, saying, "It's not that bad," usually when my pain came at an inconvenient time. "Not that bad for you maybe," I would have said if I had had the wisdom at that age. Instead, I became a disbeliever myself. I began to join the others in their determination that "It's not that bad." I learned to put my head down and resign myself to my situation without thinking about it.*

*The triple whammies of lack of opportunity to talk about my pain, the muteness and inexpressibility that I fell into when the rare opportunity did arise, and the ease of denial on the part of the observer created in me a unique web that I wove around the pain and shaped me to the core. This web was there for my survival, but like the mishmash of collagen fibers forming the imperfect reproduction of skin that is a scar, this web bound me down in places that I'm only now beginning to discover.*

*As part of my preparation for this book I recently answered a question that I will be asking you to reflect upon as well. The question is, what does pain mean to you?  Here was my answer.*

*Being in pain means that I have a parasite sucking out my lifeblood 24/7. It's not the pain that truly hurts; it's the life I'm being robbed of. The pain takes away the opportunity to show myself and the world who I truly am. There is a little kernel of the real me that peaks her head out and smiles, when things get really bad I rely on the knowledge that she's still there to get me through. The pain has put me through my own personal war zone along with the accompanying changes in my personality. My sunny disposition turns anxious, my optimism and joy turn into fear and anger, my self- love becomes guilt and loathing, my outgoing side turns quiet and shy, my love of people and social nature turn into withdrawal and feelings of isolation.*

*Being in pain means I can't take much for granted and that my trust and faith in my body has been shaken. My inalienable right as a human to free movement has been stolen. It means that ever since I was a child I've had a fantasy of taking a walkabout like the aborigines, traveling around the world with the clothes on my back and a few bucks in the bank, unencumbered, taking jobs along the way in a coffee shop to keep the money flowing. But I know that my body can't handle this so it remains a fantasy.*

*Being in pain prevents me from experiencing what I feel must be one of life's greatest pleasures, true relaxation. I imagine lying on a hammock at the beach under a palm tree, taking a nap and feeling my body melt into the cords of the rope easily and comfortably. The only sensations I have are the soft, warm tropical breezes caressing my skin and the sounds of nature in my ears. This makes me hope for a heaven so that someday I can go there and lay on that hammock. Being in pain means that I've had Owen Wilson, the actor, show up in my dreams time and time again, making me wonder why this stranger keeps entering my unconscious thoughts until I realized, " I want to be like the person he portrays on the screen, relaxed, go with the flow, happy go lucky, and successful." To know that kernel of me is like his persona, but the parasite that is pain has changed this. Being in pain means that I have to have an unshakable belief in myself and who I am even when my behavior doesn't reflect this. I have to feel the isolation of chronic pain, as there's very little chance someone without pain will have any idea about any of this, but I also have to deal with the tendency I have to shut down instead of doing the work it takes to have an honest relationship with those close to me.*

*Unlikely as it seems, this parasite that is pain has created tremendous opportunity for me to become an enriched human being. This opportunity includes the possibility of true compassion that I can offer to those around me, the opportunity to be extremely grateful for this gift we call life, the opportunity to have a real relationship with myself and others, and the opportunity to discover just how strong I can be.*

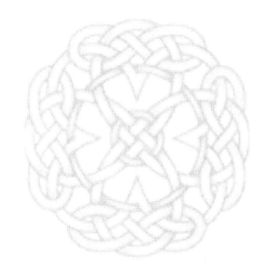

## Chapter Two:
## PAIN is a Four Letter Word

*"The world is full of suffering. It is also full of overcoming it."*

-Helen Keller

I titled this chapter *PAIN is a Four Letter Word* because there are a lot of people living in pain, myself included, who at times think it should be a swear word. I'm sure there are also a few creative people out there who have turned it into one more than once. When you live with pain for any length of time you quickly realize how it can permeate every area of your life and seemingly every pore in your body. At times you may begin to become consumed with figuring out ways to extinguish it or at least turn down the noise, and when you are not doing that you are trying to distract yourself. However, you are always acutely aware that no matter how hard you ignore pain, it is still there. Pain is like the elephant in the room, embarrassing and unsightly, but completely present.

Pain is primitive and primal and is a fact of life not only for us humans but for animals as simple as the one celled amoeba. Pain is so prevalent in the animal kingdom because it keeps us alive. People who have the rare occurrence of the inability to feel pain don't live as long as the rest of us, their body is working so hard to mop up the damage that's been created by a life without pain. But pain at certain levels can also make us want to be dead. In fact, before the discovery of general anesthesia people routinely chose death over the dreaded experience of a surgery where they would feel every cut. The surgeons in those days would come into the operating room with a bottle of whisky not only for the patient, who hopefully got first dibs, but for himself and his assistants so they could endure the agonizing screams they would be hearing over the next few hours. After anesthesia, the so called "world's most important medical discovery," came into popular use in the late nineteenth century, life expectancy went up from thirty five to fifty, over twenty five percent.[1]

Pain has many definitions. According to the American Pain Association, pain is defined as, "An unpleasant sensation that is subjective in its interpretation and has an emotional component associated with actual or potential tissue damage." More simply put, MedicineNet.com states pain is an, "Unpleasant sensation that can range from mild, localized discomfort to agony" And then there is my personal favorite from the book, *The War on Pain*, "Pain is what the patient says it is." Because pain is so elusive medical science is only beginning to truly understand it in its many forms and with this understanding is coming much improved pain management.

However, for many people there is still a long way to go. Because pain can't be seen on a biopsy, found in the bloodstream, or otherwise pinpointed through traditional medical diagnostic routes, and because it is often hard to treat, pain is frequently minimized or mishandled. Pain in rheumatoid arthritis is often treated as a peripheral issue and left up to the patient to manage on his/her own. In my long thirty-seven year history with pain, not once have I had a doctor explain pain to me or offer any tips to handle it, although it is the pain, not anything else that limits me in my everyday life. Over the course of this chapter I am going to attempt to remedy this situation by explaining what we know about how pain works in the body, talk about pain in arthritis, and then, most importantly, ways to live with pain and still have a life.

The first modern theory describing pain was introduced by Rene Descartes in the seventeenth century, a fascinating scientist and philosopher who is credited with the legacy of the mind/ body split in science. Descartes believed that pain traveled through the body along mini sensory highways that looked like threads. Amazingly, given the resources available to scientists in the 1600's, he was largely correct.

The pain pathways theory led to the idea that pain was hardwired, involving a harmful stimulus and a response. The stimulus/response theory was the accepted explanation through the 1950's. According to this theory you have an unpleasant stimulus, say a needle stick. This stimulates specialized nerve fibers called nociceptors that travel to the brain, where the harmful stimulus is registered and then sends a message back to the site and produces the sensation of pain. Nociceptors are unique nerve receptors found on the skin and in most tissues of the body. They are the first link in the chain that ends in a perception of pain. The stimulus, for example the needle stick, always produces the same response, therefore the term hardwired. How many of you think that if you took a poll of your friends everyone would report an identical experience of pain when having their blood taken? Do it the next time you go to the doctor and see what people say. You'll soon realize that the term hardwired is misleading.

In the 1960's two pioneers in the field, Patrick Wall and Ronald Melzack, furthered our knowledge about the pain experience. They described what they called the gate control theory of pain. This theory basically says that when pain signals travel through the nervous system they are controlled by chemicals that decide whether to let them in or keep them out. In certain extreme circumstances, for example the soldier who doesn't feel his injured limb until after the battle is over, the brain will bar the entry of the pain sensation until the victim is safe. Another aspect to this theory explains that pain signals travel through the same pathways as other sensations, like touch and pressure, which is why rubbing a hurt arm or leg can make it feel better.

## *The Brain in Pain*

We now know that there is a lot more to the experience of pain. A pain signal traveling to the brain goes through two relay stations deep in the brain and from there it is farmed out in three directions, each of which have specific ramifications for the perception of pain. The first stop is the cerebellum, part of the brain that is involved in movement and coordination. The cerebellum, upon being stimulated gives an urgent signal to the body to move away from the painful stimulus. The next area of the brain that is stimulated is a structure in the limbic system which regulates moods and emotions. This is where we create our emotional response to pain. Our response is based upon past experiences, coping skills, beliefs and fears surrounding the pain experience. The intensity of our emotional response will either magnify or decrease the feeling of pain. The third area that is stimulated is the frontal cortex, a portion of the brain where we do our conscious thinking. This is where there is an attempt to interpret the experience, where we ponder "Why?" Through learning, you will avoid repeating the experience.

This is a wonderful system for short-term, or acute pain when the amount of pain experienced is directly linked to the degree of injury. In chronic pain, or pain that persists, this system can actually end up backfiring. A person in chronic pain has no way to move away yet the brain is repeating this command. This ends up creating either a guarding response where the surrounding muscles tense up, leading to muscle fatigue and even more pain, or a freezing response, which is a reaction against this signal to move. One reason why exercise can be so helpful for people in chronic pain is because moving serves a need in the brain.

The emotional response is tricky in chronic pain because it can become self stimulating. In other words, past experience colors your emotional reaction to your present situation. If you are in pain long enough eventually the emotions surrounding the painful experience can start coming first and end up creating more pain. Pain will unknowingly end up changing your reality until your reality revolves around pain. If this isn't enough, the frontal cortex gets involved, begins the learning process by asking "Why?" without receiving a satisfying answer, and very soon the "Why?" can turn into "Why me?," "What's wrong with me?," etc. This useless mental exercise can quickly degrade into feelings of helplessness, hopelessness, and anxiety.

Another aspect to chronic pain is called pain centralization, or a pathologic change in the nerves and a resulting disturbance of function. It was demonstrated in 1965 by two researchers, Mendell and Wall, that when certain pain fibers found in muscles, called C fibers, were stimulated repetitively there was a progressive buildup of the response, which they termed wind-up. Wind-up happens because at least one chemical, called substance P, will migrate to the area and sensitize surrounding tissues. Substance P can diffuse over long distances without losing its effectiveness and even turn on nearby muscle groups that haven't been injured, and it stays awhile causing widespread and prolonged tenderness following tissue injury in deep muscle tissue. In some cases, the nerve endings may even fire at harmless stimulation like joint motion or light pressure. This is because, as the gate control theory demonstrated, pain fibers converge onto the same nerve ending as other nerve fibers and once sensitized this nerve ending may become confused.[2] This is when chronic pain actually loses its function and why in chronic pain there is no direct link between the injury and the

42

experience of pain. Your body may be talking to you but there's no reason it should.

Now onto rheumatoid arthritis pain. People with rheumatoid arthritis experience a combination of acute and chronic pain, sometimes at the same time. Most pain in rheumatoid arthritis is caused by stimulation of pain fibers during chronic joint inflammation. During inflammation there is an abundance of neurochemicals which can stimulate the pain fibers. The swelling also causes pain because it stimulates mechanoreceptors, substances that respond to stretch or pressure. In addition, once inflammation subsides pain often results from the altered mechanics of the joint caused by the swelling or the resulting joint destruction that has occurred.

Injury to the nervous system in arthritis occurs because repetitive pain fiber stimulation can result in central sensitization. In other words, over time, with repeated painful stimulation in the joint, nerve endings may fire more easily resulting in increased pain. Pain in rheumatoid arthritis it is so changeable and hard to put a finger on because it comes from a variety of places.

Happily for all of us, along with the new understanding of the complexity of the pain experience in the body comes improved knowledge of how best to address it. The pain experience is now seen as a series of layers. The innermost layer is the pain stimulus, then the discomfort, distress, the pain behavior, and finally the interaction with the environment. All the layers influence the experience of pain and therefore all the layers need to be addressed in order to create real change.

There is, however, a very important layer, or more accurately one that interweaves through all of them that has been left out and that is previous experience. I mentioned this earlier but I want to explain it further because I feel it is something that isn't addressed enough, especially in the context of rheumatoid arthritis, and is important to consider when examining your emotional response to the pain.

Although I can't prove it scientifically I'd bet anyone that people with rheumatoid arthritis deal with pain at a level of severity and duration that is largely unmatched in any other chronic disease category. I'll also go out on a limb and say that severe pain is a traumatic experience. Borrowing from research on post-traumatic stress disorder it is known that after a major traumatic event the physiologic response to this event can be triggered at a later date when something similar is experienced, even if it is seemingly benign.

To explain this in another way, a soldier who saw his buddy die in combat may later experience the same stress response in his body along with the feelings of panic, fear, and anxiety that he did during the actual event when he hears loud noises. Someone with arthritis who woke up one day with knees so swollen he couldn't move them, and so hot he could fry an egg on them, could  conceivably experience similar emotions such as fear, anxiety, and panic years later when he has a flare and his knees swell again. The longer your history with arthritis, the more likely this will happen and that you'll have more than one traumatic event to contend with.  If you're not careful all of this can create a tangled web wherein physical and emotional responses are triggering each other. This is what I call suffering because it layers an experience that is seemingly out of your control on top of an event or circumstance that is out of your control. A long-standing history with arthritis is an invitation to suffering.

But suffering can be avoided if you know how to do it and is imperative in living well with pain. When pain is a part of your life avoidance of suffering seems like a worthwhile goal to me.  I'm not suggesting that I can teach you how to never suffer again but I am saying that there are ways to walk through it, meet it and sidestep, or ideally transform it altogether. The first step in this process is to sit with your pain for awhile and begin to experience it without judgment.

## *Holographic Pain*

With my new understanding of pain I've come to think of pain experience as a hologram.  This multidimensional picture incorporates a physical, behavioral, and emotional experience that is happening simultaneously. In order to effectively live with pain it is important to look deeply at each aspect of this holographic experience.

Take a minute and get a pen or pencil. Then refer to the end of this chapter and fill out the Holographic Pain sheet as you read this.

Let's start with the physical symptoms.  What symptoms do you experience, along with the actual pain?  Some may include fatigue, decreased concentration and memory, muscle tension, insomnia, and gastrointestinal upset.

Next examine how the pain has changed your behavior. What activities have you decreased or stopped in the areas of work, household chores, social life, exercise, hobbies, and family activities? Think about how other people's reaction to your pain may be changing your behavior.
What feelings and thoughts do you have in response to your pain? Some common responses include anger, depression, fear, anxiety, lack of control, hopelessness, decreased self esteem, denial, or failure.

Finally, consider the question I answered at the beginning of this chapter, what does being in pain mean to you? [3]

 It is important for you to understand the impact that pain is having on your life so that you can take steps toward a meaningful life with pain and begin to transform your suffering.

## *Changing Pain-Getting Started*

Now that you have identified the far reaching effects of pain on your life, you can begin exploring ways to alleviate the pain as much as possible without having a life that revolves around it. This may take some diligence and will entail changing some of your habits but it will be well worth it.

## 1. Get to know your pain

This is a variation on acceptance of pain. Many experts in the field will tell you how important acceptance is and they will say that people who accept their pain improve more. I tend toward a slightly different idea. I accept my present reality as one that involves pain, but I leave plenty of room for the possibility that this can change for the better at any time. Accepting my pain today will immediately help to lessen it because pain has a way of fighting back when you struggle against it.

 One way to get to know your pain is by keeping a pain diary. There are two examples in the back of this chapter, the first is a diary you fill out at the end of each day and the second is one that you can use at any time throughout the day. Both will help you to put words to how you are feeling and better understand your emotions and behaviors in response to your pain. Getting to know your pain will also help you to pace your activities more efficiently.

## 2. Allow yourself to change your negative psychological reactions to pain into more helpful states of mind.

Consider this quote from Lance Armstrong, a professional bike racer who lived through stage 4 testicular cancer and went on to win seven Tour de France competitions. *"You can alter any experience with your mind- it's up to you to determine what the quality of each moment is. Concentration and belief can make the chemotherapy, no matter how sickening it is, a positive experience. It takes practice but it is possible. I used to tell myself when I threw up or when it burned so badly to urinate that the sensations represented the chemotherapy leaving my body. .. I wasn't going to dwell on whether I was going to die. There were those in medicine and those outside it that thought I would die but I chose to be around doctors and nurses who believed I could make it."*[4] Lance did what he could to remain positive during his grueling experience in part because the alternative was unthinkable. Whether throwing up really was the chemotherapy leaving his body or not is beside the point, what really mattered was that he was improving his state of mind.

It's important to remember that we are constantly framing our experiences with our thoughts, something I will describe in some detail in the chapter on stress. Examining how we respond to situations in our minds can not only help to change the stress response but will also have a positive effect on your body by increasing the body's natural pain killing endorphins. Remember that on a physiological level pain is experienced both emotionally and physically. Your emotions are just as strong at influencing the pain experience as any medicine or treatment you may find. If you are telling yourself how horrible your life is as you are receiving a massage you will continue to exacerbate the pain and minimize the positive effects of the massage. On the other hand, if you use Lance's technique and spend the time visualizing the massage rubbing the pain away, you'll enhance the effects.

A powerful way to work with pain is to explore your relationship to it. Think about:

- o *What have I done in response to my pain?*
- o How have I thought about it?
- o How does it make me feel?
- o How does it make me suffer?

Not easy questions, I know, but worthwhile ones to explore.

Once you are able to really sit with the pain and explore your relationship to it you will begin to be able to separate the actual physical pain experience and the ensuing suffering. The suffering comes about through judgment, expectation, anticipation, fear, and anxiety. All of these create and sustain negative emotional states which end up causing more pain. In the book, *The Art of Happiness,* co-written by the Dalai Lama and Howard C Cutler, MD, there is a wonderful exploration of this. Although chronic pain may seem to have no purpose, meaning can be found by contemplation of the many benefits pain has. As I said earlier in this chapter people who can't feel pain don't live very long. The disfigurements that are so common with leprosy aren't caused by the disease, but instead are caused by loss of pain sensation which creates an "utter nonchalance towards self destruction." People with leprosy have been seen to walk on exposed bones or stick their hands in a fire to retrieve something. So pain can be seen as a valuable tool. I know that if my pain didn't warn me of the inflammation in my joints I would be pushing my body well beyond its limits.

The other unfortunate thing that people with leprosy experience because of their lack of pain is a feeling of disconnect from their bodies. "Of course, I can see my hands and feet, but somehow they don't feel part of me. It feels as if they were just tools... Thus, pain not only warns us and protects us, but it unifies us." Before I learned this fact I would often lament to myself that my pain made me very aware of different body parts. My knees are constantly telling me they are there. But then I remembered falling asleep on my arm, waking up and looking at it, and not realizing it was mine. For a few moments I felt the experience of a person with leprosy and I very quickly began to appreciate the painful body that I know is mine.

Finally, in the words of the Dalai Lama is what I consider to be the most meaningful part of pain. "But anyway, I think that there is one aspect to our experience of suffering that is of vital importance. When you are aware of your pain and suffering, it helps you to develop your capacity for empathy, the capacity that allows you to relate to other people's feelings and suffering. This enhances your capacity for compassion towards others. So, as an aid in helping us to connect with others, it can be seen as having value. So, looking at suffering in these ways, our attitude may begin to change; our suffering may not be as worthless and as bad as we think."[5] Remember in the beginning of this chapter when I answered the question, "What does being in pain mean to you?" I started out describing it as a parasite that sucked out my life blood and ended up saying it creates an opportunity for me to be an enriched, compassionate human being. Is it possible that pain can be both of those things?

Working to transform your pain will uncover negative beliefs that you hold about yourself and the world that are damaging. This is a necessary step to move towards a more helpful state of mind. When you begin to write down your thoughts around pain you'll discover attitudes and assumptions, usually when you are telling yourself you "should, must, or ought to." Underneath these lie what are called core beliefs. Negative core beliefs are what generate the "should" statements you end up thinking. Let me give you an example of this.

Here is an exercise taken from a wonderful book called *Managing Pain before it Manages You* by Margaret A. Claudill, M.D.,PhD. Pretend you wake up with increased pain on a day that you had planned to visit a friend.

- What would you say to yourself?
  (These are your automatic thoughts).
- How would you feel physically?
  (This is your physical response).
- How would you feel emotionally?
  (This is your emotional response)

My first thoughts are "I need to get up and spend the day with Sara. If I don't go she'll be upset. I should be able to do this, why can't I be like a normal person and not have to deal with this pain? I'm going to be in so much pain I will have a hard time keeping up. I'm not going to be able to have fun and I'm going to be mad about this. Sara is going to be frustrated with me."

I'm feeling tense and my pain is getting worse. In the anticipation of the day I'm already mad, feeling left out, and lonely. My thoughts uncover my assumptions about the way the day is going to go and the reaction of those around me.

 If I look further into this thinking though I will uncover the core beliefs I have held, which are that people don't want to deal with my pain and that I am alone. Once I realize this is where all the anxiety is coming from, I can look into how I came up with these beliefs and begin to challenge them. Instead of believing my friend will become frustrated and upset at my pain, I can now understand this comes from my own fears and begin to release those fears. From there I can examine the problem from a more realistic perspective i.e., the fact that the pain may prevent me from carrying out the plans with my friend that I was looking forward to. Once I see the real problem I will be putting myself back in the driver's seat and increasing my control over the situation.

Another technique, created by psychologist David Burns, called the vertical arrow, can also help to uncover your negative core beliefs and fears. If what you're saying to yourself is true you can ask, "Why does this upset me?" "What's the worst thing that could happen?" Then you write out your responses to these questions. Look at your responses and ask yourself the same questions again. Drawn an arrow down and write out those answers. Keep doing this until you have uncovered the real issue.

Here is an example:
> If you wake up in pain and think to yourself, "My friend will stop asking me to do things if I keep canceling because of my pain,"

> Ask yourself, "Why does this upset me?"
> "What's the worst thing that could happen?"
> - "It upsets me because I like to be true to my word, and now I'm an unreliable person."
> - "I hate to be left out."
> - "I'll be isolated and alone."

**Bingo. The real issue. Fear of being alone.**

Once you become adept at reframing your thoughts you'll realize that you are actually suffering less, which is the ultimate goal.

A final word from the Dalai Lama,

> "If you have fear of some pain or suffering, you should examine whether there is anything you can do about it. If you can, there is no need to worry about it. If you cannot do anything, then there is also no need to worry." Enough said.

## 3. Break any habits that reinforce the pain

A good portion of our behavior is conditioned, more than most people would like to admit, and sometimes behavior that is the result of pain can end up reinforcing it. In other words, if you avoid the stairs because it hurts to walk up them you will end up with a deconditioned body and more pain. If you withdraw into yourself instead of engaging with friends and family, you may end up isolated and depressed. The way you communicate your pain to others can also end up reinforcing it. I'm going to discuss in depth the delicate balance of communication and rheumatoid arthritis later on in this book but for now it is important to think about how your loved ones treat your pain. They are constantly walking a fine line between ignoring it and the tendency to do too much or overprotect you. And if you aren't honest with yourself and open about your needs with others your behavior and your loved one's response may become an uncomfortable dance.

Again, let me explain. Most of my life I had the tendency to be stoic. It was a matter of pride with me never to complain or seem weak. I would keep going until I literally couldn't move anymore and then I'd be in crisis mode and I'd become the center of attention because of my pain. While I was being stoic on the outside, on the inside I'd be watching the people around me, blissfully unaware of my pain, and I'd become upset at their inattention to my needs. When my body finally broke down and I got the attention I'd been craving all along I'd feel a huge wave of relief that I didn't have to carry this huge load on my own anymore. I'd secretly be lapping up all the care and attention I finally was receiving from my loved ones.

The obvious problem with this is that I could have avoided crisis mode entirely if I had thrown my pride out the window and asked for what I needed to begin with. The last thing you want to do is have a chimpanzee jump on the gorilla on your back and that is exactly what bad habits will become. So to prevent this from happening refer to the holographic pain worksheet that you filled out earlier and look at the section on behavior. Which behaviors listed are actually reinforcing your pain? Once you've identified them you'll have a place to start creating change.

## 4. Create a pain plan

Because rheumatoid arthritis causes a variety of types of pain, it is useful to have a variety of pain control methods in your arsenal. Working with your thoughts and emotions and breaking bad habits will by far have the most powerful and far reaching effects on your quality of life in the long run, but sometimes you need relief NOW. Quite understandable I'd say. Thankfully there are many options you have at your disposal for quick relief.

Here is a list of options that I've used successfully:

*Heat* can be used on painful areas alone or in combination with stretching. The reason heat works to decrease pain is because it reduces muscle spasms, relaxes surrounding tissues and increases flexibility. Heat can be applied in the form of hot packs, hot water bottles, and in clinical settings, ultrasound treatments.

*Cold* decreases circulation to the area and can reduce inflammation especially when it's caused by overdoing it.[6]
The question is when to apply heat and when to use cold. Both will decrease your pain but they work differently on the painful area so the rule to follow in most cases is to use cold when your joints are very hot and inflamed and heat when the pain is caused by muscle tightness and you need to promote relaxation in the area.

*Gentle movement* helps on many levels. I discussed earlier that pain creates a need in the brain to move. Gentle movement will not only fill that need but will release tight muscles, improve your posture, and improve your mood. Gentle movement can come in the form of simple stretches, tai chi, chi gung, walking, or yoga among other things. The key is gentle. Movement that is fast or forced may cause increased tightness and spasm.

*Orthotics* include splints, compression stockings, and ace bandages. The goal with these devices is to provide stability to joints that have become unstable either through inflammation or joint changes and provide rest to painful joints thereby decreasing pain. Splints are usually obtained by consulting an occupational therapist who will be able to fit the splint to you and teach you proper use. One common splint is a resting hand splint which puts your hand in a functional position and rests it there while you sleep. There are also finger splints which help support fingers that have overstretched tendons. One company, The Silver Ring Splint Company, makes finger splints that look like rings and these splints can be quite attractive. In fact, when I had one I frequently got compliments on my cool "ring." The best thing to do is to consult an occupational therapist who will evaluate your need for splints and fabricate the best splints for your needs.

**Compression stockings** and gloves help the pain by actually decreasing the swelling in your joints. You can experiment with simple compression gloves from your local pharmacy but once again you need to consult an occupational therapist to get custom made garments which are the most effective. Wearing gloves at night can significantly help with morning stiffness and pain and my personal experience with wearing the stockings has been amazing. I wear them during the winter and not only do I keep my legs warm, I also experience a night and day difference on days when my knees are swollen. They are worth every penny in my opinion. Ace bandages are inexpensive and easiest to get since you just need to go to your local grocery store. Once you have one play with it on your ankles and hands. Don't put it on so tight you lose circulation and be careful if you try one on your elbow or knee because it may increase swelling in the hands or feet if you leave it on too long. The best way to use an ace bandage is during activity, taking it off after you finish whatever you are doing.

*Massage* is a term that encompasses quite a variety of techniques. Probably the most common technique is Swedish massage, which is a kneading of the soft tissues and can improve pain by increasing circulation, relaxing muscles, improving sleep, and possibly increasing the release of endorphins. The important thing though is that it feels good! If you have the resources finding a good massage therapist is well worth it as is experimenting with the more specialized forms of massage such as myofascial release, rolfing, cranial sacral therapy, shiatsu, and deep tissue. Myofascial release works on the superficial fascia layer that creates a sheath around muscles and organs. Rolfing is a comprehensive, full body technique that works all the layers of tissue from the fascia to the deep muscle tissue, and its goal is to restore correct movement, posture, and function, thereby relieving pain. Cranial sacral therapy works on the fluid that baths our cranium and vertebrae all the way down to your pelvis. There is a delicate rhythm that moves this fluid created by our breathing and movement and working on this rhythm can improve our nervous system and pain. Shiatsu is a Japanese form of massage that works on meridians and acupuncture points, improving the energy flow in the body. Finally, deep tissue work goes straight to the deep layer of muscle and is effective for people who are very tight from overuse, sports, or long term pain issues.

*TENS* , otherwise known as Transcutaneous Electrical Nerve Stimulation, is electrotherapy based upon the gate control theory of pain. Stimulating nerves will inhibit the pain response from reaching the brain and will also stimulate the nervous system to produce endorphins, our natural opoids.[7] TENS treatment is something you can pursue with your physical or occupational therapist and may help you get through pain flare ups. There is a more sophisticated form of TENS, called ETPS, or electrical therapy point stimulation, that I am a huge fan of. It combines myofascial release, acupuncture points, and osteopathic theory to address acute and chronic pain issues.

*Analgesics* include over the counter and prescription drugs, topical creams, as well as herbs. Pain is something to discuss with your doctor and hopefully you will be able to come away confident with your knowledge of the costs and benefits of using drugs for pain. You can also go to a pain center where you will find specialists in the field. Topical creams are an easy route you can explore on your own and can be very effective for muscle pain. When you are looking for a cream be sure to read the label and find the cream that has the highest menthol and salicylate levels because they are going to be what relieves the pain. Creams that have capsaicin, the active ingredient in hot chili pepper, have been shown to decrease levels of substance P, a chemical that increases pain and inflammation. The catch with these creams is that they really burn especially if you get the area warm. The last thing you want to do is to rub one of these creams on and then go out and exercise. I know this from an experience that I never care to repeat. The official word is that your body will eventually accommodate to the cream and stop burning but I've never been able to tolerate it that long. After my experience with exercise and accidently touching my eyes after applying the cream I decided that the pain wasn't that bad!

 If you want to pursue a more natural approach you can investigate the use of herbs and supplements. Stick to quality nutritional companies so you know that you are actually getting what you see on the label and don't try too much at once, otherwise you'll have no idea what works. This is something you'll have to do a bit of trial and error with; then again that's what the doctor is doing when he or she tries you on a new drug.

**Homeopathic medicines** are widely used in Europe by medical practitioners. In the United States you have to delve into the alternative arena to find someone who can advise you. You can also do a bit of research and self treat by trying remedies that match your symptoms as much as possible. You want to dissolve homeopathics under your tongue and avoid eating or drinking around twenty to thirty minutes before or after you take them.

Here's a list of herbs and homeopathic medicines that treat pain: (Not inclusive)

| Homeopathic Medicines | Herbs |
|---|---|
| Rhus Tox | Ginger |
| Sulphur | Turmeric |
| Arnica | Fish Oils |
| Kali Mur | Bromelain |
| Ruta Graveolens | Cat's Claw |
| Rhododendron | Angelica |
| Calcarea Carbonica | Chamomile |

*Acupuncture* is practiced widely in Asia and has been around much longer than Western medicine. A licensed acupuncturist will place very small needles in your skin on points that correspond to energy pathways called meridians. The meridians travel through our body just like our blood vessels and when stimulated will balance your energy flow and can boost the body's ability to heal itself. The needles rarely hurt going in and once in you shouldn't be able to feel them at all.

*Saunas* are used in Europe and Asia for pain and are starting to be found more in the States. You can purchase a sauna for your home and although it will be an investment, it is one that has alleviated severe pain for me. At times I've hobbled into my sauna and walked out. The key is to use a far infrared sauna, not the traditional hot stone sauna. Far infrared heat is part of the sun's invisible spectrum and penetrates human tissue over one and a half inches to easily reach muscles and joint tissue. Unlike hot air saunas that heat up to 180-235 degrees, far infrared saunas will provide benefits at a much lower temperature, 104-130 degrees, and therefore are much safer and well tolerated. Saunas are great for many reasons, not only do they decrease pain, they provide a workout for your heart muscle because heart rate and cardiac output are increased, increase your metabolism which helps burn calories and control weight, and provide direct elimination of toxins through the skin.

*Aromatherapy* is the use of the essential oil of plants, through inhalation or absorption. Like many so called alternative therapies, it has been around since ancient Greece and was rediscovered in the early twentieth century in France. Aromatherapy is widely used in Europe and Japan for a variety of ailments. Inhalation is the safest method to start with because there is no risk of irritation to the skin and when you inhale essential oils you are immediately affecting the deep brain which regulates mood, emotion, and hormone release so this can have a powerful effect. Absorbing essential oils through the skin carries them into your bloodstream and you can do this by adding a few drops into a bath or putting them into a carrier oil and using them for massage. The important things to remember are never to use an oil full strength on the body, if applying one to the skin testing it on a small area to see if you are reactive, avoid touching your eyes after contact with the oil, only use therapeutic grade oils not synthetic or perfume oils, and remember to avoid any oil that comes from a plant you know you are allergic to.[8]

The best way to obtain essential oils is to find a practitioner who has training in the area and discuss your needs with them. You can do this by asking at your local health food store, looking in the phone book, or finding a young living essential oil representative in your area. Young living is one company that I know has quality oils and also trains its representatives well.

**Here's a list of essential oils that have analgesic or anti inflammatory properties:** (This list isn't inclusive)

| Eucalyptus | Clove | Peppermint |
|---|---|---|
| Lavender[1] | Ginger | Pine |
| Jasmine | Chamomile | Sage |

*Biofeedback* is a form of complementary medicine that utilizes a machine to measure a person's heart rate, galvanic skin response (sweating), blood pressure, brain waves, and/or muscle tension in order to give them real time information about their bodily processes. It was developed in the 1960's by a group of researchers who were interested in accessing the autonomic nervous system, which until that time had been thought to be out of reach of conscious control. It can be used to alter the body's innate reactions to pain. Biofeedback creates a mirror so you can see your automatic responses and then consciously alter the responses that reinforce or increase the pain. One type of biofeedback, EMG biofeedback, will give you real time data that will show you where you which muscles are tightening around the pain when you move and then you can learn to consciously relax those muscles so you don't create more pain. EEG biofeedback will work with the brain's response to pain and help you to relax around the pain. Biofeedback is a valuable tool and you can find a certified practitioner by looking at the website for the

---

[1] One of two oils you can use straight on your skin.

Biofeedback Certification Institute of America, www.BCIA.org, and going to the find a practitioner section.

*Distraction* is always an option anytime, anywhere. It's the mental version of the gate control theory, meaning that if you are focusing on a funny movie or beautiful sunset you won't be focusing on your throbbing finger. The best forms of distraction involve something funny or absorbing in a pleasurable way. Arts and crafts have been a great form of distraction for me. When I tore a ligament in my knee I spent a good chunk of my recovery period painting t shirts. It was fun, kept my mind off the pain and disappointment I felt, I learned something new, and I had gifts for people so I felt I was doing something useful with my time. Use distraction consciously throughout the day when you need a break from the pain.

This list is by no means complete. I could write a whole book just on this one area but let this be a jumping off point for you to start. The key is to try different things and become familiar with which techniques work best for different types of pain. Then when you have a bad pain day you'll be ready to head it off before it becomes overwhelming. At the end of this chapter I have included a Pain Day Plan worksheet for you to fill out. Write down options you have at your disposal using this list, other ideas you may have, and other sections in this chapter, and keep it handy for the day you need it.

## 5. Identify a pain support network

Whether you know it or not, your pain affects those close to you too and if they get involved in the coping skills you are cultivating they are less likely to undermine them or feel depressed and anxious about what you are going through. If you've ever been on the other side of severe illness you'll quickly understand how difficult it can be. Knowing what to say, when to say it, when to intervene and offer help and when to let the other person work it out on their own, these are questions that have no definitive answers and may change at any time. Because your loved ones struggle with these issues every single day it's important to consider their needs and still meet your own.

One good way to do this is to have an extended network of people who you can rely on to give you the support you need so you never overburden one person. Even if you have eliminated entirely all your negative reactions to pain, broken all your pain reinforcing habits, and diligently followed through with your pain plan, there still is no getting around the fact that pain is a negative sensory experience and being bombarded with unpleasant sensations for much of your life will take its toll. The truth is that you'll need help some days physically, some days emotionally, and some days both.

Through the years I've been extremely lucky to have many really good friends who have literally saved my sanity and my joints. I'm eternally grateful for this and I'm also very careful not to rely too heavily on one person no matter who they are. The exception to that rule (and you know there has to be one!) is my Mom. I know that she has borne the burden of being on the receiving end of the majority of the days when I have nothing left and all I want to do is cry, rant, rave, and generally feel sorry for myself. I also know that has created a lot of anxiety for her, especially when I was living far away and she wasn't seeing that eighty percent of the time I was doing just fine. When I realized what I was doing and how it affected her I began to make a point of reaching out when I was doing great, not just using her as venting board and this created a lot more balance in our relationship.

Creating a pain support network also involves calling upon people's strengths and not expecting them to be able to be something they aren't. Some people are really talented at seeing the amusing and hilarious in situations but won't be as good at sitting with you handing you tissues as you have a good cry. Some people will be excellent at solving problems that come up and others will be there when there are physical chores that are too difficult for you. Take some time right now, go to the end of this chapter, and fill out the pain support network form. You'll find that creating and using your support network will change all of your relationships for the better.

## 6. How to deal with relapse - keep trying

In living with a disease that involves experiencing more pain in a year than most people will in a lifetime it is easy to get discouraged. This is especially true when you have a period of time with less or no pain and then it comes back. When this happens it's easy to begin to feel that all your effort to create a better life and control the pain and disease was for nothing. It's easy to think that the disease controls you not the other way around. It's easy to begin to feel sorry for yourself. It's really easy until you realize that by thinking this way you've actually made your life really hard.

It's vitally important to remember that you will have good days and you will have bad days. This is your life. You don't have to like it; you do have to accept it for what it is. You have to accept yourself, your life, your pain, even on the days when you don't. Accept your self -judgment, accept your mistakes, accept your negative thinking and then move on. You may think you've taken two steps forward and two steps back, but life isn't a straight line, it's a spiral. Everything spirals back to where it started eventually, this you don't have a choice in. What you do choose is how you meet it when it does. Learn to do it a bit better each time and you will create a well lived life. This you can be proud of. When you are in the midst of a relapse do the best you can to take care of yourself, as you would any cherished loved one until the recovery comes, because it will.

## Chapter Two Worksheets

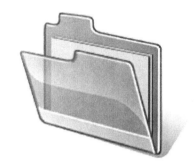

- Pain Diary 1
- Pain Diary 2
- Holographic Pain
- Pain Day Plan
- Pain Scale
- Letting go of Suffering
- Uncovering Core Beliefs
- Pain Support Network

# PAIN DIARY 1

Where did I feel pain today?_____

_____

_____

_____

_____

Describe it:_____

_____

_____

_____

_____

How bad was it at its worst (1-10)?_____

Did it change with activity? If so, describe the activity:_____

_____

_____

_____

_____

Was it better at any time of day? If so, when?_____

_____

_____

Did anything help the pain?_____

_____

_____

_____

_____

Did anything make the pain worse? _____

_____

_____

_____

_____

# PAIN DIARY 2

Date:_____          Time:_____

What you are doing?_____
_____
_____
_____
_____

Pain sensation: (1-10) _____

Describe physical sensation: _____
_____
_____
_____

Describe self talk and mood that followed:_____
_____
_____
_____
_____

Describe emotional response:_____
_____
_____
_____
_____

Can you re-frame thoughts: _____
_____
_____
_____
_____

Action taken: _____
_____
_____
_____

Pain sensation after action taken: _____
_____
_____
_____

# HOLOGRAPHIC PAIN

What physical symptoms do you experience, along with the pain: _____

_____

_____

_____

_____

_____

_____

_____

_____

What activities have you changed, decreased, or stopped because of the pain?
How do other people's reactions influence your behavior? _____

_____

_____

_____

_____

_____

_____

_____

_____

_____

_____

_____

_____

_____

What feelings or thoughts do you have in response your pain? _____

_____

_____

_____

_____

_____

_____

_____

_____

_____

_____

_____

Adapted from *Managing Pain Before It Manages You,* by Margaret Claudill MD, Phd

# WHAT DOES BEING IN PAIN MEAN TO ME?

# PAIN DAY PLAN

I have many resources to get me through this day. I am confident that this will pass; my body is more resilient than I know. I have people that love me, activities that I enjoy, compassion for myself, and patience. *(Add your own thoughts here)*

_____

_____

_____

_____

_____

_____

_____

_____

_____

_____

_____

_____

My Options for Pain Relief

1. _____

2. _____

3. _____

4. _____

5. _____

6. _____

7. _____

8. _____

9. _____

10. _____

# PAIN SCALE

**0** - I have no pain

**1** - I barely notice my pain

**2** - It's not a bother

**3** - It is there but I can control it

**4** - My pain is starting to impinge on my daily activities

**5** - My pain isn't constant and I can't get relief

**6** - My pain is constant and I can't get relief

**7** - My pain consumes me

**8** - It's REALLY bad

**9** - I'd like to lose consciousness right now!

**10** - I am in the worst pain imaginable

1 _____ 10

# LETTING GO OF SUFFERING

What have I done in response to my pain? _____
_____
_____
_____
_____
_____
_____

How have I thought about it? _____
_____
_____
_____
_____
_____
_____
_____

**How does it make me feel?** _____
_____
_____
_____
_____
_____
_____

How does it make me suffer? _____
_____
_____
_____
_____
_____

Can I allow it to just happen, can I let go of suffering? _____
_____
_____
_____
_____

# UNCOVERING CORE BELIEFS

Describe a situation when you experienced increased pain: _____

_____
_____
_____
_____

What were you thinking? _____

_____
_____
_____
_____

What were you feeling physically? _____

_____
_____
_____
_____

What were you feeling emotionally? _____

_____
_____
_____
_____

Examine your thoughts and emotions and list any negative core beliefs:

_____
_____
_____
_____
_____
_____
_____
_____

# PAIN SUPPORT NETWORK

Who makes me laugh and can see the humor in situations? _____

_____

_____

_____

_____

_____

Who can help me physically? _____

_____

_____

_____

_____

_____

Who can help me to solve problems? _____

_____

_____

_____

_____

_____

Who will bring me comfort when I'm feeling down? _____

_____

_____

_____

_____

_____

Who can provide emotional support? _____

_____

_____

_____

_____

_____

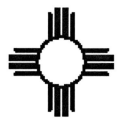

*There are certain memories that stick with you forever and you can't help but wonder why. For me one of those memories is when I was in fourth grade. I was walking home from school and trying to count how many worries I had. I came up with ten. Earlier I had heard that most adults worry about seven things every day, in one of those "good thing you're still a kid" speeches. It surprised me to learn that kids were supposed to be carefree because I felt anything but and I decided to count my worries to see how I compared to the average adult.*

*At the time no one would have guessed I existed in this state of mind. I was voted the happiest camper at summer camp during grade school which shocked me because I spent the entire time worrying about how I was going to keep up with the other kids. Camp meant swimming, hikes, and games with a bunch of kids who cried if their shins got scratched. All of my physical energy was spent keeping up with these kids and all of my mental energy was spent figuring out how to hide my pain.*

*My parents had all of their four kids enrolled in sports and for me that meant the first whiff of spring would bring a pit in my stomach along with the first flowers. Spring meant softball season and another season of grinning and bearing it. This attitude eventually became so ingrained in me that I began to live the motto "no pain, no gain." I even chose this saying for my high school yearbook picture.*

*In fact, the "no pain no gain" attitude did help me make it through some very tough days. I remember being in high school, first period biology, sitting there dreading the end of class because it meant I was heading to gym and at 8:30 in the morning I was still really stiff. The term morning stiffness was not in my vocabulary, though. In those days they didn't talk to kids about those kinds of things. Going to the doctor meant getting seven vials of blood taken, having him take my blood pressure, move my joints, and talk to my Mom. He always seemed satisfied with my answer of "fine" when he asked how I was feeling.*

*Since nobody talked about the arthritis, I ended up thinking it was a horrible family secret that I must do my part to keep. I can't tell you how many "sprained ankles" I had as a kid (code for my ankle hurt so I was limping). My parents were ill-equipped to handle a kid like me. They had three other children to take care of, had no experience with chronic health issues, and thirty five years ago medicine was in kindergarten when it came to arthritis let alone chronic pain in children. As far as emotions and arthritis, journals were pointing to an association with arthritis and "histrionic personality". Not that very helpful to say the least. Given my situation, denial seemed an obvious approach. That and numbing myself through sheer willpower and the infamous "no pain no gain" saying.*

*The other coping technique I came up with was even less helpful. At one point I decided I was fighting a civil war inside my body and I needed to subdue it. The unhappy consequence of this was the anger an internal war causes, layered on top of the anxiety I felt the rest of the time, worrying about how to* keep up.  This metaphor joined my motto and proceeded to wreak havoc in my life.  In deciding that my body was fighting a civil war, I became my own worst enemy.

When you are at war you get angry, and when there is no one to be angry at, you're likely to turn your anger inward and start using it on yourself.  I became quite an internal taskmaster.  I had no tolerance for my own body's discomfort.  I would go on hikes and end up with bleeding blisters that took months to heal.  I'd go skiing with my family and see how long I could last with ski boots on my feet, wanting to scream from the pain and I'd tell myself that it made me ski better.   I'd carry around my bottle of aspirin and, just like Dr. House on television I'd chug my 4 pills every 4 hours and keep going.  Taking long bike rides with 70 ounces of water on my skinny back, I'd get frustrated when my shoulders hurt later.  I'd never allow myself to cry; crying meant I was losing the war.  These days I wish I'd cry more.

Which brings me to another experience that I know I share with other people with arthritis, the disconnect you end up feeling toward your body.  At a young age I started to treat certain parts of my body as if they were separate people.  My right ankle was the little sister I protected, my left ankle was the proverbial "red headed step child" that better behave or else, my stomach was a guest I tried hard to please and often complained loudly at me, especially after the ulcer I got from all that aspirin.  My answer to an uncomfortable body was to leave it.  I'd go to another place in my head and become Robin Hood's sidekick or Casper the Friendly Ghost.  Now that I think of it, Casper was an interesting choice since he doesn't even have a body to contend with.

My young self was trying to handle something that could break grown men by the thousands, and then I hit puberty. How was I going to handle adulthood when being a kid was so hard? As per usual, I had a bumpy ride. My second menstrual cycle never stopped. I happened to be on a ski vacation with two families and started bleeding so much that I was using a whole box of pads a day. I had no idea this wasn't normal, and the women in the house just thought I was being inept when I woke up with blood all over my sheets. Seven days later I wasn't bleeding so much, but it was hard to walk up the stairs because I was so tired. A trip to the doctor ended up as five days in the hospital getting blood transfusions as they tried to discover what was wrong.

My answer to the pesky problem of puberty was to stop it. I lost weight and kept losing until I ended up back in a hospital, this time for six months. I wish I could say that during my time in the hospital I had a wise psychologist who helped me uncover the roots of my self destruction like Robin Williams in "Good Will Hunting." Instead, I had a pipe smoking psychiatrist who patronized me and I ended up with six months of literal silence. Here's how our daily sessions would go. Dr. X: "So anything new? Me: "Nope." Then sixty minutes of quiet. I often wonder what he wrote in my chart, "The child appears mute, but she can say the word nope." After six months I decided I wanted out by my birthday so I gained enough weight to be let out of the hospital and ended up with another thing to blame myself for and that I didn't talk about. Years later I was *able to delve into that period of my life and realized that the anorexia was another form of disassociation, just like leaving my uncomfortable body to become Casper the Friendly Ghost. It also occurred to me that disassociation was a perfectly reasonable survival technique during certain times in my life, but I turned this skill on its face and used it to harm myself.*

*Which leads me to the reason for this heartfelt rambling-stress. The subject of this chapter. Stress, which is all about how you handle it. Stress, as Wayne Dyer says, "There is no such thing as stress, only people with stressful thoughts."*

*What does stress have to do with my autobiography? You really need to ask yourself that question. Stress has everything to do with your autobiography. As you will see in the next chapter, stress is largely subjective, dependent upon your perception, and your perception begins to form when you are young. In my case, the techniques I came up with to survive my childhood ended up creating and perpetuating the harmful stress I encountered later in life. It took going through the worst flare up in my life for me to stare my stress in the face and see it for what it was, negativity that was draining me of my very life. Going back many years ago when I counted my ten worries (the bicycle drill at school, walking on the sand at the beach, playing four-square at Beth's house.....), I now see the truth of that day. Living with a chronic disease means that you have a lot to contend with and a lot on your mind. If you don't make a commitment to yourself, a vow that you will be your own best friend through it all, learn and practice ways to handle the stress that comes up, it can drown you.*

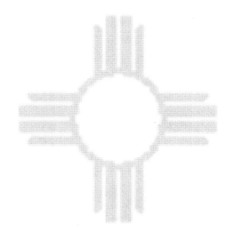

## Chapter Three:
What's Stress Got to do with It?

*"I've had a number of terrible things happen to me and some of them have actually occurred."*
*--Mark Twain*

Stress is everywhere you look.  On the freeway people swerve around you to get to their destination thirty seconds earlier. Stress is created by security and delays at the airport, deadlines at work, obligations at home. When you are living with rheumatoid arthritis, there is also the physical stress of constant pain. We are surrounded by it.

Unfortunately, the amount of stress you experience can affect more than just how harried you feel- it can also contribute to the onset and continuation of RA symptoms. Rheumatoid arthritis is a stress-related disease which means that RA and stress are connected. This chapter will help you to understand how stress affects your body and how these effects can influence your RA.

Let's begin with the definition of stress. Stress is *"The perception of physical or psychological threat and the perception that the individual's responses are inadequate to cope with that threat."* The key word here is *perception*, and the key concept is that stress is a very personal experience.  One individual may become overwhelmed and anxious about the idea of public speaking while his neighbor finds the idea to be challenging and exciting.

 In any individual stress creates a cascade of events involving a whole body response. We all have a "stress circuit" that is activated with a signal from the body (our perception).  This signal travels to a structure in the brain called the hypothalamus, which immediately begins a series of events leading to hormones being released from the adrenal glands.

All of this activity occurs within milliseconds and results in a state of hyper-arousal which has traditionally been called the fight-or-flight response.  This fight-or-flight response results in a racing heart, dilated pupils, dilation and constriction of blood vessels to allow for blood flow to the large muscles, release of glucose into the bloodstream for immediate energy, increased muscle tension, an increase in endorphins which are natural painkilling substances, an increase in immune cells, a decrease in digestion, a decrease in reproductive hormones, and the activation of the limbic system, our emotional center deep in the brain.

## *The Hare and the Tortoise*

This response was ingeniously designed for our survival. Think of the man who is able to lift a huge boulder to free a trapped child, or someone who is able to jump out of the way of a truck that doesn't see him. During these events we need energy and blood for our large muscles to work well, we need to be hyper alert and attentive and we need our immune system to be ready to take care of any injuries may sustain during the event. All of our resources are directed towards taking care of this immediate threat.

In the book *The Hare and the Tortoise, Culture, Biology, and Nature,* author David Barash makes the argument that the speed of biological change, like the image of the plodding tortoise, is steady and slow, whereas the speed of social change, like the feisty hare, is rapid. This creates a discontinuity between how we live and our comfort zone. Although multi-tasking has become the norm for most of us, our brains don't learn well or retain memories as accurately if it has to focus on multiple things at once. In fact, a good portion of the brain has the job of deciding what to attend to and what to ignore.

For eons societies were made up of small extended family groups where we lived, worked and socialized. This means that the stress response evolved when the world we lived in looked a lot different. The pace of life was slow, punctuated by short, time-limited events that were dangerous and often threatened survival. Picture a woman with her young children 100,000 years ago, gathering fresh berries in the Spring, when a hungry bear comes out of nowhere. The fight or flight response would be very handy at a time like this. Now picture the woman today, driving her children to school, late for work, when one of her kids pipes up and says that he needs to bring cupcakes to school. The stress response will hinder, not help, her ability to handle this situation. Keep in mind the concept of the *Hare and the Tortoise* as I describe in more detail the short and long-term effects of stress on our bodies and how this relates to RA.

## *Brain, Body, Stress*

Because the stress response has been so essential for survival, the emotional brain, or limbic system, is very important in our response to stress. Having an emotion attached to an event helps us to remember it and hopefully avoid it later. The limbic system is made up of two deep brain structures, the amygdala, which is small and almond shaped, and the hippocampus, which is shaped like a banana. The amygdala receives input consciously and unconsciously during perceived threatening encounters, like being chased by a bear, and is important in storing fearful memories. The stronger the emotional response, the stronger the memory will be and severe trauma will cause the amagdala to be triggered more easily the next time a stress occurs. The hippocampus is important in providing context for the threatening event. That way the stress response won't be triggered if the bear is in a zoo, only if you see it when you are picking berries.

However, over time, stress changes the structure of both the hippocampus, which shrinks, and the amygdala, which grows. The amygdala is more likely to be triggered unconsciously while the hippocampus becomes less able to modulate this response by providing context. If you live with chronic stress you may have a limbic system that is unconsciously triggering your body to produce stress hormones and you can develop damage to that area. This very situation has been shown to be true in diabetic rodents who show elevated stress hormones and damage to the hippocampus. Vietnam veterans with post-traumatic stress disorder have been shown to have on average an 8% loss in the size of their hippocampus.

Stress also suppresses the release of reproductive hormones, including testosterone, estrogen, and progesterone. This makes sense if you are being chased by a bear, but in our modern world chronic stress can result in decreased menstruation and infertility. In fact, women with high cortisol levels have three times as many miscarriages.

During a stressful event, digestion is not a priority and our body turns down the release of stomach acid and intestinal secretions. Over time, this can lead to a number of digestive maladies.

The immune system on the other hand, needs to be ready to act. During stressful events mast cells break down and release histamine and cytokines which are substances that increase the inflammatory response. With prolonged stress however, an individuals' immune response becomes less effective, resulting in increased susceptibility to disease, or oddly enough, autoimmunity.

Growth hormone can be affected as well. During acute stress, growth hormone is released in large quantities. But over time, this hormone becomes depleted, which can be especially detrimental to children. Children in orphanages who don't receive nurturing fail to grow. This quickly reverses itself if they are placed into a loving home.

Who isn't concerned about being trim? Stress can contribute to weight gain because the stress hormone cortisol releases glucose into the bloodstream for immediate energy. Over time however, this promotes fat deposits that can contribute to the onset of type 2 diabetes and cardiovascular disease.

And finally, I need to mention the connection between stress and mood. During a stressful event endorphins, our body's natural painkillers, course through our system and cause euphoria. We need this feeling so that we can actually believe it's possible to lift a boulder off a trapped child. However, that feeling of euphoria doesn't last, and over time can turn into depression and anxiety. People diagnosed with major depression have higher levels of stress hormones in their system. All of this information tells us two things: chronic stress has an adverse effect on the body and can result in disease.

## *Good Stress?*

Wait, what about good stress? Is some stress helpful? Does good stress really exist or is it just a myth? The answer is that good stress does exist, and there's a specific word for it, "eustress," Eu meaning well or good. Eustress is a helpful during challenging, stimulating, and most importantly, time-limited events. Think of exams, public speaking, or sporting events. This is completely different from the kind of stress I've been describing which is distress. Then the question becomes, how does one tell the difference?

The determining factor in deciding if stress is good or bad comes down to one thing: whether you have the ability to recover after a stressful event or whether your body continues to be activating its stress circuitry. This is the key question to ask yourself when undergoing stress. The answer is dependent upon your previous history with stress, your genetic heritage, your present reality, and your perception of the stressful event.

Let's start with genetics. Within a given population there will be a continuum. Some people will be especially vulnerable to turning on their stress circuit at the drop of the hat, while others are more like the stereotypical surfer dudes who are able to remain calm while all the Chicken Little's are running around them. In the midst of this continuum there are people who can turn on their stress circuit but have a hard time turning it off, and people who stress response is halfhearted. All of these situations can be partially related to a genetic heritage but, like most genetically related disorders genes are only part of the story. There needs to be a triggering event or events in the environment for genes to express themselves. This is where our previous history with stress comes in and where the story gets interesting.

## *Your Stress Story*

From the time we begin life in our mother's womb until adolescence (some say even longer), our nervous system demonstrates a lot of plasticity, meaning it is changeable because it is still being formed. This means that at a young age we are especially vulnerable to trauma.

Trauma can create a situation that permanently alters our stress circuitry, especially in genetically vulnerable people, which can influence your tendency towards diseases like rheumatoid arthritis.

Let me explain further.

Remember the limbic system, our emotional brain? And the amygdala, whose job it is to respond to fearful events and remember them? The amygdala is activated anytime there is a potential threat to us and early in life, as the amygdala is still being formed, it isn't as accurate at recognizing real threats or modulating its response. Think of a rattlesnake. You don't want to meet a young one in a dark alley because if a young snake bites you it's liable to inject you with all the venom it has. This is because it's still refining this technique and is not very good at gauging how much venom to release during a threatening encounter. As this snake gets older, it will become better at this skill and will be able to assess the situation more accurately. An older snake won't bite as readily and will only use as much venom as is absolutely necessary and no more.

Back to our amygdala. When we're young we are constantly monitoring our environment for perceived threats and when we encounter a situation we see as threatening the amygdala will respond strongly. The part of the brain that can provide context to a threatening situation is not yet developed enough to be discerning and allow us to respond appropriately. An example of this we've all experienced is watching a child whose bottle gets taken away. In a matter of moments they are screaming and crying as if they'll never drink again because for all they know they won't.

If we grow up in a nurturing, loving environment, we won't be bombarding our amygdala and activating our stress circuit. But if our early upbringing is less than ideal our young, unrefined amygdala will be training our brain to become hyper-vigilant through its repeated activation and strong response to our scary environment. This has been shown to be true with people who have a history of childhood sexual abuse or trauma, as well as children whose maternal figure left them at a young age. These groups of people have a higher likelihood of exhibiting abnormalities relating to their stress circuit later on in life.

Earlier I discussed how long-term stress can change different systems in the body. The important thing to keep in mind is that the effects of periods of stress can be cumulative. This means that the longer your body spends in distress, even if these episodes are years apart, and especially if the distress occurred during childhood, the higher the likelihood you'll end up with a stress-related disease like rheumatoid arthritis.

The body can only exist in a state of distress for so long before problems develop. We all have a biological tolerance for stress and when we surpass it we will begin to suffer physiological breakdown and inevitably end up with disease.

Consider the next graph:

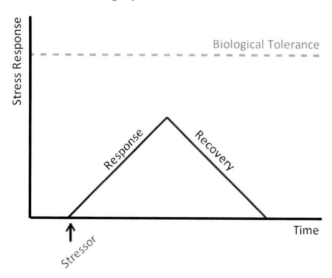

This is a healthy reaction to stress. You have a whole body response, followed by a period of recovery during which time we are able to return to baseline, our normal healthy state.

Now consider these:

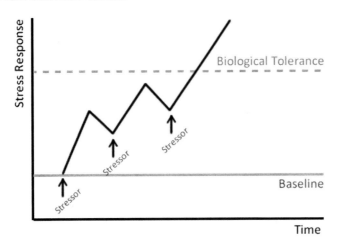

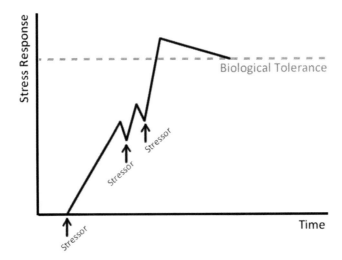

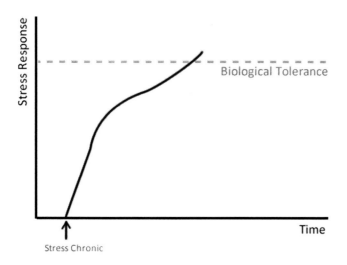

In the first scenario, you see someone who starts out at a stress level that is higher than normal.  Let's say for the sake of example that this is because she developed hyper-vigilance at a young age because she grew up in a home with parents who spent more time fighting than parenting. Notice that after each stressful event, even with recovery time, she doesn't return to her already elevated baseline. This could be because she has a genetic heritage that makes her body inefficient at turning off her stress circuit. The other possibility is that the first stressor was so significant that it began to affect how she perceived her world. Perhaps stressor number one was a relationship that soured.  Her boyfriend, who at first seemed to be so loving and supportive, lost his job and began to criticize her for every little thing she did. She is smart enough to end it, but now she begins to worry a lot.  The stress of her relationship triggered memories of her past experience and unconsciously she now returns to childhood when her hyper-vigilance helped her stay out of the way of her parents.  Unfortunately, soon after her breakup she gets into a fender-bender that ends up costing her a lot of money.  To top it all off, just like a bad country song, her dog dies.  The cumulative effect of these events, added to her return to hyper-vigilance has created a situation that exceeds her biological tolerance for handling stress and she ends up with anxiety disorder, and eventually rheumatoid arthritis.

On to graph number two. This person, we'll call him Joe, starts out at a normal baseline state. Life is good. Joe has led an average life without any significant problems in his past. Then, along comes stressor number one. His father dies suddenly. Very soon after the death of his father, distracted by his grief, he falls off a ladder when he's trying to clean out the gutter at his parents' home. He lands on his arm and breaks it. This ends up costing a lot of money because, as a self-employed plumber he depends on both his hands to work. The health insurance he purchased only covered half the cost of his emergency room visit. Joe has learned the hard way about the saying, "When it rains, it pours". Within the space of a few weeks his stress level has skyrocketed and pushed him well above his biological tolerance. Poor old average Joe ends up with severe insomnia and six months later, hypertension.

In the last graph our poor fellow starts out at a normal baseline stress level. One day while at work as a UPS driver, he delivers an especially heavy box and ends up injuring his low back. He now has pain on a daily basis. The stressor, his back pain, is the same but the unremitting nature of the stressor creates a situation where his stress circuit continues to be continuously activated without time for recovery. This poor fellow has never had to deal with significant pain before, and as a result has no idea how to handle it. His doctor is no help, other than handing out pain medication and because he's not the most emotionally expressive guy, he retreats from his family and friends. This poor fellow quickly moves past his biological tolerance and ends up not only with chronic pain, but also insulin resistant diabetes.

These three scenarios have two things in common; repeated stress resulted in a dysregulation of the stress response and eventually disease.

There is another scenario though that is very relevant to rheumatoid arthritis and this is the possibility that, when stressed, a person's physiological response isn't strong enough. I mentioned this earlier when I talked about the genetic variability in our response to stress. This maladaptive stress response is created when the adrenals don't produce enough cortisol in response to stress and as a result other players in the stress system overcompensate by becoming hyperactive. Termed burn-out, this has been implicated in rheumatoid arthritis, fibromyalgia, chronic fatigue syndrome, and seasonal affective disorder. In fact, people with rheumatoid arthritis who've had their cortisol levels measured during an acute flare usually demonstrate lower levels than would be expected and desirable.

Back to my question about how stress turns into distress. We've talked about genetics and our past history with stress. Now, let's discuss your present reality. How much stress are you dealing with in this moment in time? As someone living with rheumatoid arthritis what is important to understand is that you have an undercurrent of physical stress going on in your body most of the time so your baseline will start out higher. These stressors may include but are not limited to: physical pain, inflammation (this is not a relaxed state internally), poorer sleep quality as well as all of the activities surrounding managing the disease. You may be familiar with the Holmes and Rahe Stress Scale. It was developed in 1970 by two psychiatrists who came up with 43 stressful life events that correlated positively with the onset of illness. You can use this scale to rate your risk for illness.

The Holmes Rahe scale is a good place to start but it won't tell you the whole story. An example I use to demonstrate why is moving. Undoubtedly there will be some stress associated with any move, but the experience is hugely variable depending upon whether you are excited about the move, if you feel it's a positive step, the conditions surrounding it, (did you just get divorced or a new job, BIG difference), etc. This leads me to the last thing to consider, your perception of the event.

I've saved this for last because this is the most important factor in stress. And, as it happens, the only thing you have control over here.

## *The Power of Perspective*

How we perceive each event in our lives creates the shape of our life. Consider the following quotes,

> *"We are what we think "*                              *- Buddha*

*"We don't see things as they are, we see things as we are."*
*- The Talmud*

*"The eye is the lamp of the body, so if your eye is good, your whole body will be full of light; But if your eye is bad, your whole body will be full of darkness."*
*- Matthew 6:22*

If we look at these quotes and take them to heart we quickly realize just how important perception is. It sounds easy to say, "Just think positively," but I know that it never quite works that way. This is especially true when you've gone through trying circumstances. Sometimes the worst does happen. And when the worst has happened to you it's harder to keep your thoughts away from "What if?"

If you've taken a medicine and ended up with negative side effects, the next time it's going to be harder to get excited about trying something new. If you've been the victim of a medical mistake it's harder to give yourself over to the care of a doctor and maintaining the assumption that he or she will take care of you properly. If you were abused at some time in your life it makes sense to become more aware, less trusting. And we all know about the "Once bitten, twice shy" syndrome when it comes to matters of the heart. One heartbreak is all it can take to make someone gun shy for quite awhile.

Understanding this we can work with it. Thoughts come up automatically, seemingly from nowhere, but are actually composed of our habits and experiences along with our belief systems. Many of our automatic thoughts were formed in childhood and really have no relevance to us as adults, but because they've become ingrained into our consciousness it's hard to shake them. It's important to know that thoughts alone can create stress, but if we can start looking at our thoughts and re-framing the ones that don't serve us we literally will change our lives.

Let's begin re-framing some negative thoughts.
1. Think of a stressful situation you have, or have had.
2. Now, list how you felt physically as a result of this stress.
3. List how you felt emotionally as a result of this stress.
4. Write down the thoughts you recall having had as a result of this stress.
5. Now, examine these thoughts. Are they in any way distorted, exaggerated, or illogical?
6. If so, replace the thoughts with ones that are more realistic and positive.
7. How would you like to feel?
8. List the positive emotions that go along with the new thoughts.

Here's a list to start:
*Awareness, Awe, Acceptance, Abundance, Accountability, Appreciation, Aspiration, Balance, Constancy, Clarity, Commitment, Cooperation, Courage, Compassion, Creativity, Confidence, Determination, Depth, Discipline, Detachment, Dignity, Discernment, Ease, Equanimity, Enthusiasm, Excellence, Faith, Friendship, Forgiveness, Flexibility, Freedom, Fearlessness, Fulfillment, Gentleness, Grace, Generosity, Growth, Gratitude, Hope, Harmony, Honesty, Inspiration, Integrity, Intuition, Individuality, Joy, Kinship, Kindness, Learning, Loyalty, Leadership, Love, Mastery, Noble, Openness, Oneness, Patience, Peace of mind, Perseverance, Positivity, Power, Purity, Purpose, Respect, Responsibility, Restraint, Serenity, Service, Stillness, Stability, Support, Strength, Surrender, Striving, Tolerance, Transformation, Trust, Truth, Understanding, Will, Willingness, Vitality, Worthiness, Wisdom*

This technique was developed in the 1970's by a doctor named Aaron Beck and he coined it Cognitive Therapy. The basic principles of this technique are that our thoughts create our moods and emotions. When people are depressed or anxious their thoughts are primarily negative, and negative thoughts almost always contain distortions that are irrational. Cognitive Behavioral Therapy has been proven repeatedly throughout the years to be very effective for a wide range of issues including anxiety, phobias, chronic pain, depression, and arthritis.[9]

One thing this technique is so good at is helping you to watch your thoughts and discover their origin.

> *"The thought manifests as the word.*
> *The word manifests as the deed.*
> *The deed develops into habit.*
> *And the habit hardens into character.*
> *So watch the thought and its ways with care!!"*
> *-Ann Webster*

Perception is so important because it can turn pain into suffering, misfortune into angst, and chronic disease into powerlessness. On the other hand, it can also turn threat into challenge, chronic disease into commitment, pain into compassion, and powerlessness into control, ending up creating an immense well of internal resiliency.

Given the power of perspective we also need to acknowledge the reality that stress is a part of our everyday lives. As I've mentioned before, living with rheumatoid arthritis is physically stressful on our bodies. Pile on top of this everyday life (in a typical day the stress response is elicited on average 50 times) and you'll soon realize that learning ways to counteract these stresses would be a very good idea. As a person with RA, you need to learn stress buffering techniques and you need to incorporate them into your everyday life.

I'm going to pretend that I'm starting from scratch. I know what stress does to the body, and I want to counteract those effects. Stress tenses our muscles, makes us breathe rapidly and shallowly, our hearts beat faster and our minds race, creating feelings of danger and threat, eventually leaving only feelings of depression and anxiety. Is there anything that I could possibly do that has the opposite effect?

## *Free, Fun, Relaxation*

Why, yes there is! And it happens to be free, fun, and something that's been done in some form worldwide for thousands of years. (No, not sex!) It is a state of mind that has been named by Herbert Benson, MD,

"The Relaxation Response". The actual definition is: "A state of relaxed, passive attention to a repetitive or absorbing stimulus that turns off the "inner dialogue" thereby decreasing the arousal of the sympathetic nervous system." Something that monks, nuns, yogis, tai chi masters, the Dalai Lama, and many others spend a good chunk of their lives practicing. Over 30 years ago, Herbert Benson and a team of researchers got permission to go to Tibet and study a group of Tibetan monks. He was the first Westerner to ever get the privilege to witness some very ancient and private spiritual practices. He was able to come home with some amazing data demonstrating that people who make a lifestyle of spending time in the relaxation response end up changing their brains. They increase the thickness of the prefrontal cortex, an area of the brain that is important in reasoning and problem solving and increase the size of the hypothalamus, which as you recall, shrinks during prolonged stress. Years of research has further shown that when a person is in this state, their breath slows down and becomes deeper, heart rate and blood pressure decrease, and slow brain waves which is conducive to healing and relaxation.

Research has also shown that with increased regular practice, the relaxation response can improve quality of life in people with a variety of health problems including heart disease, anxiety, depression, rheumatoid arthritis, cancer, and post traumatic stress disorder.

There are four ingredients to eliciting the relaxation response. The first is a *relaxing environment*. You may want to listen to relaxing music or practice in a complete silence, but the important part is no phone, television, or other distractions that will bring your attention to the outside world. The second is *focused attention.* You may want to focus on an object, a word, a feeling, a prayer, an affirmation, an image of yourself as healed, or a sound. You are directing your attention to clear the mind and in doing so are focusing on your inner, not outer world. The third is a *passive attitude.* It is important not to judge, and when thoughts wander or feelings come into the consciousness, as they will, you allow them to pass noticing, not judging them. This is the most crucial aspect of the relaxation response and often the most challenging. By simply letting your thoughts come and go like waves, you'll begin to realize that's what they are, waves on top of a vast sea of calm. Eventually, you may be able to recognize painful sensations that way too. The fourth and final element is a *comfortable position*. For most people with arthritis that will be lying down, but you can elicit the relaxation response during movement. When people are practicing tai chi, chi gung, and some forms of yoga they are in the relaxation response for much of the time.

Two questions may have come up by now. First, is the relaxation response just another fancy word for meditation? And secondly, what if I'm in too much pain to relax? The answer to the first question is no; meditation is one way to get there, but there are many more choices. We'll discuss the second question later but for now let's learn how to truly relax.

***Diaphragmatic breathing*** is the simple act of learning to breathe deeply. It is very powerful and can be done many times throughout the day. Breathing with the diaphragm helps to release muscular tension, massage the internal organs, calm thoughts, and turn off the stress response. For people who feel they aren't able to set aside time daily to practice the relaxation response, short sessions of deep breathing and counting, or saying an affirmation can still have a very positive effect. Deep breathing is easy to learn, and is a natural process that we all are born knowing. As we get older, talking, habitual postures, and yes, stress, creates a situation where we breathe deeply very rarely. Paying attention to the breath and letting it lengthen is all it takes to get back into this good habit. Here's how: sit in a chair with your feet flat on the floor, or lie down. Place one hand on your abdomen, just above the navel and the other hand on your chest. Now, take a breath in through the nose. Image your lungs are a balloon that inflates as you breathe in and feel your abdomen rise up into your hand. After the belly fully expands you will feel your other hand move as your chest begins to fill with air. Once the lungs are full, you begin the out-breath by pursing your lips and pretending you are blowing out a candle. As you breathe out your top hand will move toward your body first, followed by your bottom hand as your lungs fully deflate. Pairing this with breath counting or an affirmation (In breath, "I am", out breath "relaxed," "at peace," "healed," etc.) creates the relaxation response.

***Imagery /Visualization*** is another natural process that we do all the time when we plan our day, think about future events, or daydream. Using this technique begins with breathing, inviting the body to relax, and then visualizing a place of healing in your mind. Using all your senses you visualize this place while you feel the experience of healing. You can ask questions or make a request while you are there, and it is amazing what you will find out. In my opinion, the power of visualization is extremely underutilized in medicine. Luckily, you don't need a prescription for this, just a curious mind! When you are starting out it may be helpful to find someone who can guide you or you can buy an imagery CD. There are many choices out there, my favorites happen to be by Bernie Seigel MD and Dr. Andrew Weil, the important thing is to experiment and have fun.

***Progressive Muscle Relaxation*** is a form of relaxation developed in the 1920's by an American physician named Edmund Jacobson. This technique is interesting because it will increase your awareness of your bodily sensations. It takes less than twenty minutes and involves systematically tensing and releasing your major muscle groups, starting with your facial muscles and gradually moving down to your feet. The muscles to focus on include; face, neck and shoulders, chest, abdomen, left arm, left forearm, left hand, right arm, right forearm, right hand, left leg, left lower leg, left foot, right leg, right lower leg, right foot. Begin by lying down, getting comfortable, and taking a few deep, diaphragmatic breaths. Then, inhale and tense the muscles in your face for about eight seconds. Exhale, and relax those muscles fully. Then, move to the neck and shoulders and so on. As you practice this technique, you may begin to notice feelings that come up when you are tensing or releasing your muscles. Eventually, the goal is to be able to notice when your muscles are tensing, or when you are having feelings associated with tension throughout your day, and then to stop this tendency by immediately relaxing that area. This is a great skill to develop, especially when you are in pain much of the time. With chronic pain comes the natural tendency to guard the painful area and this will decrease blood flow, causing more pain. Speaking of pain, when you are practicing this technique, avoid tensing to the point of significant pain. The last thing you want to do is strain your muscles or joints.

*Autogenic Training* is a form of self-hypnosis developed by a German neurologist named Johann Schultz. In the 1930's he combined his knowledge of brain research and his interest in hypnosis, to come up with a way that patients could "self-regulate" in order to induce hypnosis on themselves. Autogenic actually means self regulation, and the idea is to help you train your nervous system to be more flexible and relaxed. There are many variations to this technique which ideally, should be practiced daily for at least six months to gain full benefit. Since this is a bit more advanced, I suggest if you are interested in autogenic training to look for a professional who can guide you until you feel comfortable doing it on your own, or buying an autogenic training CD. Here's a sample of what a typical session would involve. You begin by getting comfortable, breathing deeply, and saying to yourself "My breathing is easy and smooth." Then, focus on your dominant arm and say to yourself, "My right (left) arm is warm and heavy" six times. Turning your attention away from your arm, say to yourself, "I am quiet and relaxed," "My heartbeat is calm and strong," six times. Return to your breathing and say, "It breathes me" six times. Finally, focusing on your stomach, imagine sun rays settling there and say to yourself "Warmth is radiating over my stomach." To end, continue to breathe deeply and make a couple of fists, move you arms gently, and open your eyes. There are many other variations on this theme, but the idea with them all is to use your thoughts to guide your body to a relaxed and comfortable state.
**Biofeedback** is something I discussed in the last chapter on pain. It can be extremely helpful with altering the stress response as well. The fight-or-flight response is turned on by part of the autonomic nervous system and biofeedback can access this. During a biofeedback session, you will be practicing some of the techniques I already described and simultaneously you will be receiving information about how your body is responding. It can increase the learning curve for inducing the relaxation response

*Tai Chi/Qigong/Yoga* are all forms of exercise that incorporate gentle movements of the body along with breathing and visualization. They can be considered moving meditations because they focus and calm the mind. Each has a unique origin. Yoga has its roots in spiritual practice, with the name yoga literally meaning "union" or "to yoke." Tai Chi was originally an internal martial art associated with Taoism. Qigong is associated with traditional Chinese medicine. The world's largest medicineless hospital, called Huaxia Zhineng Qigong Clinic and Training Center operated from 1988-2001, when it was closed down for political reasons. This clinic used a 5,000 year old method of qigong with the people who came to be treated and remarkably had a 94.4% healing rate (15% cured, 38% very effective, and 42% effective.) Even more remarkable was that most of the people who came were there because traditional approaches hadn't worked.

All three of these gentle exercises have been practiced for thousands of years and are now becoming well known in the United States. I would highly recommend trying one or more of them not only to reach the relaxation response but because they have tremendous benefits for pain, balance, strength, and range of motion. Be careful to find a gentle form of yoga though; some types of yoga may strain joints too much.

***Repetitive Movement*** involves shifting focus when you exercise to your breath or rhythm of your movement. Combining the rhythmic nature of exercise and focusing your thoughts can be very conducive to relaxation. You'll also begin to notice where your thoughts usually take you, which can be very informative.

***Mindfulness*** is the basic practice of awareness. We spend so much of our time on automatic pilot that sometimes we don't even remember what we just did. Ever put your glasses down and then forget where they are ten minutes later? That isn't early Alzheimer's, it's not being mindful. Mindfulness keeps us in the present moment and away from our conditioned thoughts, anchored in the past or future. It can be done anytime, anywhere, and all it takes is shifting your focus to the present. A simple mindfulness exercise is called the *raisin experiment*, introduced by Jon Kabat Zinn MD, who founded the Center for Mindfulness in Medicine at University of Massachusetts Medical School. You take one raisin, put it in the palm of your hand, look at it; notice its shape, size, texture, and all the details you never noticed before. Then place it on your tongue and begin to taste. Leave it there for a few moments before beginning to slowly chew and, finally, swallow. That simple experiment will clearly demonstrate to most people that they normally eat raisins without truly tasting them or even noticing what they are doing. Mindfulness will also increase your awareness of your automatic thoughts, which can help you shift them. Mindfulness enriches your experience of life by helping you to stop, look, listen, and pay attention, instead of just going through the motions.

This short list will hopefully give you some ideas about how to incorporate relaxation into your life. The important thing is to choose one that works for you and your lifestyle.

## *Pain as a Teacher*

Now, let's discuss the second question, "What if I'm in too much pain to relax?" This is a very valid question that doesn't have a simple answer. Feeling relaxed can be a very rare experience when you are in pain, which can make attempting meditation or any other mindful practice very frustrating. I once attended a weekend workshop on meditation led by a Tibetan Lama. We were meditating sitting in chairs, and the minutes seemed like hours to me because I was so uncomfortable. Later when he took questions I stood up and asked how to meditate through pain. He just looked at me, and I saw his eyes soften as he said, "This is a very difficult situation."

Later I read some of the Dalai Lama's teachings and I found a more satisfying answer. According to the Dalai Lama, pain and suffering are two different things. Pain is a physical sensation while suffering is the mental angst we place on top of it. In our society we have come to believe pain is an affliction that needs to be eradicated. In actuality, pain is a part of the experience of living. When we start to believe that we have to be comfortable all the time it places an unrealistic expectation that creates irrational thinking. Physical pain is accompanied by the real affliction, negative thoughts and emotions such as anger, envy, fear, or anxiety.

Using pain as a teacher when you practice relaxation will ultimately help you gain tremendous insight into your own unhealthy thought patterns. Practicing relaxation and examining the thoughts that come up when you begin to experience pain can teach you about your fears and beliefs. With practice, you will be able to let them go and replace them with more helpful states of mind. So, someone who has pain as their constant companion may be in a difficult situation, but also has the opportunity to practice the ultimate goal, peace of mind. This is a tool that people who live a more physically comfortable existence don't have. Stop thinking about pain as an affliction and start to think of pain as a way forward. As the Dalai Lama says in his book *Ethics For A New Millennium,* "Gaining insight into our own negativity is a lifelong task, and one which is capable of almost infinite refinement. But unless we undertake it, we will be unable to see where to make the necessary changes in our life."

Pain can then become, like our negative thoughts, the waves that sit on top of a sea of calm. I'm not in any way trying to downplay the effect pain has on a person's everyday existence, I'm only pointing to the fact that adding negative thoughts to the pain will be detrimental to your life. When you are practicing relaxation, start by getting as comfortable as possible and when pain comes up, breath into it, examine any uncomfortable feelings that arise, and then let them go. It took me many years to realize that by fighting pain I was feeding it. Now I relax into it and find that it stops being so loud.

So far I've talked about perception and relaxation as ways to buffer stress. There is another very important piece of this puzzle, a piece that is so important I'm devoting a whole chapter to it. That piece is social support. I probably don't even need to mention all the research showing that people with rheumatoid arthritis who are satisfied with their support network have less active disease and significantly less psychological distress, or the higher risk of death for heart attack victims that don't feel that they have support. It is pretty obvious to most people that having support makes you feel good and feeling alone increases your stress level. Unfortunately, our world today can be a very lonely place even for people who have a support network. People are busier than ever, emails and phone calls have replaced tea time, even people who live in the same house end up needing to schedule time together. The answer to this is to make time together a priority. Get together with your friends and family and have fun, laugh, cry, tease each other, exchange massages, and know that you are doing your body and soul good.

Here we are in this country desperately trying to discover the solution to the rise in every chronic disease category by looking at the Mediterranean diet, why French women don't get fat, exactly how many minutes you should exercise every day, 10,000 steps a day or 12,000, and in reality the question we should be asking ourselves is, "How many belly laughs have I shared with someone today?" People who love you will be able to speak for you when you are feeling so low that the well of positive thoughts has run dry. When there is nothing left to say they will be there to give you a hug, knowing that you will be there for them when their day comes.

*"Everything can be taken from a man but….the last of human freedoms to choose one's attitude in any given set of circumstances, to choose one's way"*

*"When we are no longer able to change a situation we are challenged to change ourselves."-Victor Frankl*

Victor Frankl, a psychiatrist who ended up in a concentration camp in World War Two II, is one of my heroes. His experiences there formed the basis for logotherapy, a new approach to psychotherapy which theorized that a man's primary motivational force in life is his search for meaning. By answering for and taking responsibility for one's life, this meaning is born. Simply stated, in the words of Nietzsche, "He who has a why to live for can endure almost any how." I strongly believe that one important challenge for someone with rheumatoid arthritis is to find that meaning. Without a core of meaning and the belief in oneself that comes with it, the challenges of rheumatoid arthritis will become overwhelming. And the stress that you feel as a result of the disease can, as I said earlier in this chapter, drown you. Use what you've learned in this chapter to deepen your insight, change your perspective, create new habits, and most of all, commit to yourself to find your driving purpose and live it every day.

# *Chapter Three Worksheets*

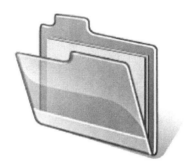

- Stress History Worksheet
- Stress Buster Worksheet
- Thought Log
- Remembers the Real You
- The ABC's of Me

# STRESS HISTORY WORKSHEET

List any traumas you endured at a young age: (abuse, upheaval, loss of a parent or

care giver, injury/illness, etc.) _____

_____

_____

_____

_____

_____

_____

_____

List all significant stressors you have endured as an adult: _____

_____

_____

_____

_____

_____

_____

_____

_____

_____

List any stress related physical symptoms you have had and the time period:
(Insomnia, lack of menses, digestive upset, weight gain/loss, increase in
colds/flu/infections, autoimmune diseases): _____

_____

_____

_____

_____

List any mental symptoms that you have had related to stress:  (anxiety, depression,

hyper-vigilance): _____

_____

_____

_____

_____

# STRESS BUSTER WORKSHEET

List current stressors: _____

_____

_____

_____

_____

_____

_____

_____

Check all stress buffers that will help with your current stressors:

____Cognitive re-structuring     ____Time with a supportive friend

____Vertical arrow technique     ____ Exercise

____Progressive muscle relaxation     ____Reading

____Advantage/Disadvantage list     ____Meditation

____Tai chi/ Chi gung/ Yoga     ____Aromatherapy

____Music     ____Deep breathing

____Relaxation/Imagery     ____Writing/Journaling

Write down affirmations that will help you to change your perspective about your stress: _____

_____

_____

_____

_____

_____

_____

_____

_____

_____

_____

_____

_____

_____

**Place these affirmations on a card and look at them often.**
**This is who you really are!**

# List all daily activities by placing them on this scale:

**Negative** ------------------------------**Neutral**----------------------------**Positive**

(I really hate doing this activity)                                              (I LOVE doing this!)

Your scale should tip largely to the right. What can you do to make this happen?

_____

_____

_____

_____

_____

_____

# THOUGHT LOG

**Stressful Event:** _____

Physical signs: (List how you feel physically as a result of the stress.)

_____
_____
_____
_____

Emotions: (List how you feel emotionally as a result of this stress.)

_____
_____
_____
_____

Automatic thoughts: (Write down the thoughts you recall having as a result of this stress.)

_____
_____
_____
_____

Cognitive distortions: (Identify the distortions in each negative thought)

_____
_____
_____
_____

Positive thoughts: (Substitute more realistic and positive thoughts, "What do you want?")

_____
_____
_____
_____

Positive emotions: (How do you feel as a result of these new positive thoughts?)

_____
_____
_____
_____

# REMEMBERING THE REAL YOU

Who were you when you were twelve? What were your favourite things to do, see, or experience?_____

_____

_____

_____

_____

_____

_____

_____

_____

_____

_____

_____

_____

_____

Remember the child you were you still lives inside you today. How can you bring this child back into your life? _____

_____

_____

_____

_____

_____

_____

_____

_____

_____

_____

_____

_____

_____

_____

_____

_____

_____

# THE ABC'S OF ME

You are many wonderful things.  Using each letter of the alphabet, list positive qualities that you have. Use this list whenever you need a pick- me-up. You can do this for others too, what a gift!

A _____

B _____

C _____

D _____

E _____

F _____

G _____

I _____

J _____

K _____

L _____

M _____

N _____

O _____

P _____

Q _____

R _____

S _____

T _____

U _____

V _____

W _____

X _____

Y _____

Z _____

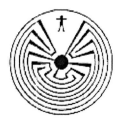

*Because I've had rheumatoid arthritis all of my conscious life I never went through a period of questioning how I got it. It was always there, a part of me. It wasn't until the arthritis went quiet and then came back with a vengeance that I started delving into what causes this intense pain and swelling. Unfortunately, I came up with more questions than answers.*

*We are only beginning to understand how the cells of the immune system work and what happens when they become so confused that they begin to attack our healthy cells. There are many plausible causes: infection, faulty genes, toxins in the environment, allergies, and stress, to name a few. Most likely there is more than one combination of factors that can lead to RA. And because there are so many unknowns regarding the causes of RA - much less a cure - the questions then become, When you have rheumatoid arthritis, do you really need to try to figure out what caused it? What will knowing do for you if there is no cure? If it will all be conjecture anyway?*

*For me, knowing what caused my RA isn't as important as knowing what I can do now to manage the symptoms and hopefully coax it into remission. This can help me today, with or without the 20/20 vision of hindsight available to me. The ultimate goal and golden rule is to dampen the flames of inflammation, to keep putting cogs in the wheel of this vicious cycle until it stops. The theories that are being tossed around about the cause of rheumatoid arthritis and the knowledge we have about inflammation help us to know where to put those cogs. Understanding the details about your immune system will help you to know what your doctor is trying to do when he or she suggests a certain treatment strategy or medication to you. Knowing the details of how inflammation works in the body will help you to ask the right questions of yourself and others as you go through the process of putting out the fire in your joints. You will be able to guide the process with more confidence and become an active member of your healing team. Nobody has all the answers, only educated guesses, and knowing what questions to ask may actually be the key. This chapter goes into a lot of detail, but only skims the surface of everything that is being looked at with regard to the origins and management of RA. Think of this chapter as a buffet, take what you want, need, and feel good knowing, and don't worry about the rest. You can always come back for more later.*

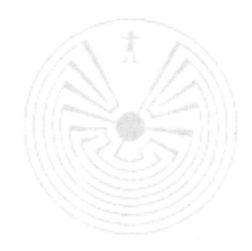

# Chapter Four:
## Inside Arthritis

*"The doctor of the future will give no medicine,
but will interest his patients in the care of human
frame, and in the cause and prevention of
disease."*

*- T. A. Edison*

What causes rheumatoid arthritis? What makes it worse? What makes it better? Why does my rheumatoid arthritis affect me differently than other people I know with the disease? Why does one drug work and not another? These are common, understandable questions you may have already posed to your doctor.  If so, you may have heard, "Well now, that's the million-dollar question!"  So, without knowing the answers to all of these questions, how does one effectively treat the disease? To me, **THIS** is the million-dollar question.

In this chapter, I'm going to describe the major players in the immune system and how medical research into the immune system over the years has affected thinking about rheumatoid arthritis, as well as treatment approaches. I'm going to explain inflammation, the hallmark of rheumatoid arthritis, and how it can go awry. I'll explain what affected joints look like and also touch on other systems that can affect inflammation.  All this information will help you better understand the questions we all pose and what various RA treatments are aiming to do.

Arthritis is over a hundred different diseases. What the diseases in this huge category all have in common is joint (arth) inflammation (itis). The tendency towards arthritis is something we humans share in common with all large bodied land animals. The fossil record has even revealed arthritis in prehistoric humans. Arthritis remedies are found in the folk medicine of just about every society in the world. Given the length of time people have been experiencing arthritis we have had disappointing results trying to get rid of it. Despite all the advances of modern medicine the numbers of people with arthritis keeps rising. Thirty years ago one in seven people had arthritis in this country, now the number is closer to one in three.

Rheumatoid arthritis is the second most common type next to osteoarthritis. Diagnosing rheumatoid arthritis can be difficult and often takes months, if not years because the symptoms are so variable. The reason for this is that rheumatoid arthritis is systemic, meaning it affects not only the joints but the entire body. People with rheumatoid arthritis can experience a myriad of symptoms including gastrointestinal problems, flu- like symptoms that don't go away, weight loss, extreme fatigue, anemia, osteoporosis, changes in sensation, and skin reactions, to name just a few.

The hallmark of rheumatoid arthritis is severe swelling of the joints, usually in a symmetrical fashion. For unknown reasons, if one ankle develops swelling it will usually be on the person's dominant side and then the other side will follow. This applies to any joint that becomes involved. When a joint becomes swollen, especially early on, it will feel hot to the touch, painful, and may have a reddish tint. This is because there is a lot of activity going on inside the joint which is a result of inflammation.

Inflammation is the body's normal response to injury or infection and is mobilized by the immune system. When an injury or infection occurs in the body, specialized immune system cells gather at the site to rid the body of any foreign matter, including cells and molecules that are dangerous. These immune system cells produce factors to repair wounds, clot the blood, and fight any infective agents. During the process this area becomes inflamed and some healthy tissue can be injured. Normally this process is brief and as soon as the infection is contained, inflammation subsides.

Let's use the example of a paper cut. Broken skin has allowed bacteria to enter. Within seconds the invader has been detected and blood rushes to the area. The capillaries in the surrounding tissues become more permeable so that fluid and immune system cells can easily enter. These cells surround the bacteria, create chemical messages that signal other cells to join them, and soon they destroy, contain, and remove the harmful bacteria. Your paper cut started out as a thin red line, became more red and swollen, pus may have formed, and then the skin heals and the area returns to normal.[10]

In rheumatoid arthritis and in any chronic inflammatory disease the immune system mobilizes, creates inflammation, but fails to subside and destruction of healthy tissue occurs. Once the joint has arthritis it becomes enlarged, bones and cartilage erode, the lining of the joint is thickened, and tendons and ligaments become stretched as they pass over this enlarged joint. The alignment of the joint itself is altered. When this happens in the joint it alters the precisely designed structural system that enables us to move and function efficiently. The result is pain, fatigue, and the wear and tear that happens when tendons move across joints that are misaligned.

All flexible joints are lined with something called synovium. Synovium produces synovial fluid, a clear substance that lubricates and nourishes the joint. A person with rheumatoid arthritis experiences inflammation of the synovium. The synovial lining becomes three to ten times thicker and infiltrated with immune system cells that produce inflammation. The fluid that is supposed to nourish joint structures also becomes filled with inflammatory cells and plasma. Extra fluid rushes in, stays there because the capillaries are more permeable letting in more and more fluid, and the joint becomes puffy. Cartilage, which cushions the end of bones and is normally very resilient, begins to degrade and become dehydrated. Nearby bone erodes. Tendons and muscles that cross the joint become stretched and damaged.[11]

If you think of the joint as a pulley system you can imagine how altering mechanics can alter function. Designed to lift heavy loads, pulleys are comprised of a sturdy frame, a rope or belt, and a wheel that smoothly guides the rope attached to the load. It is an extremely efficient system when designed correctly. In our bodies a pulley system creates movement around joints. The sturdy frame is our skeletal system, the wheel is the joint, and the rope is our tendons or muscles. Changing the size of the wheel will change the way the rope moves and either make movement less efficient, damage surrounding structures, or prevent movement altogether.

In rheumatoid arthritis one very common deformity of the fingers is called a boutenniere deformity. This deformity occurs when the pulley system that extends the middle finger joint is altered. First, the middle finger joint becomes inflamed making the joint, or the wheel of the pulley system, bigger. Then the tendon, or rope, becomes overstretched to the point that it no longer can glide smoothly over the joint. The sheath that holds the tendon in its proper location ruptures and the tendon falls to the side of the finger. Now, when you try to lift the finger, the middle joint stays bent. Eventually the tendon shortens and the middle finger joint become fixed in this position. Once this happens your movement patterns will have to shift in order to perform the same tasks and the joints surrounding the altered one will have more stress placed on them. This is an example of how sustained inflammation can create permanent alterations in the structure and function of your joints, the movement of your body, and possibly set you up for pain that is not just isolated to your affected joints.

Now that we have an understanding of inflammation, let's talk about the cells that create it, specifically the cells of the immune system.

## *Welcome to the Immune System*

To say that the immune system is a mind-boggling complex is an understatement. Specialized cells in our immune system are so diverse that they can recognize almost any molecule in the universe. Only very recently have medical researchers begun to understand its basic workings, although clues that such a system existed became apparent centuries ago with the discovery of the smallpox vaccine by Edward Jenner in the 1790s. Louis Pasteur expanded on this in the 1800's and developed the germ theory of disease. Soon, more vaccines were created including those for anthrax, rabies, and diphtheria.

By the turn of the century there were two schools of thought about how the immune system functions. On one side were the scientists who believed that immunity was found in the "humors" or fluids in the body. On the other side were those that proposed a cellular source, specific cells that ate invaders. It wasn't until well into the 1900's that it became known that both theories were true and not until the 1960's that modern immunology was born.[12]

Our basic knowledge of how the immune system works has evolved considerably over the past fifty years. In the 1950's the presence of antibodies, small proteins that bind to regions of foreign substances called antigens, were all that were known about immune responses. This is when the term autoimmune disease was born and autoimmunity became the prevailing theory to explain rheumatoid arthritis because people with RA were found to have antibodies against their own healthy cells. Rheumatoid arthritis was thought to be a disease in which the body attacks itself due to an overactive immune system. This explanation continued to dominate prevailing thinking and treatment for years to come and has only recently begun to change. In the 1960s, it was discovered that T cells and B cells communicate with each other. In the 1980s, immune cells were discovered to release molecules called cytokines, which help to control the immune response. Over 100 cytokines are now known to exist and many of them have overlapping functions. In the 1990s, a new T cell called regulatory T cells, were discovered. [13]

These discoveries began to shed light on possible mechanisms of action in rheumatoid arthritis but unfortunately, until recently had little or no effect on treatment options for people with the disease. Before the millennium, aspirin was one of only a few drugs developed specifically for arthritis. All of the other drugs that treated arthritis were either discovered to work by accident or developed for different purposes and later found to benefit people with arthritis. Many of these drugs were used for decades before a general understanding of how they were affecting the disease was known. Widespread suppression of the immune system was the only treatment available that demonstrated effectiveness for more severe episodes of arthritis and this, of course, came with many side effects.

There were three classes of drugs used to treat arthritis: non-steroidal anti-inflammatories, corticosteroids, and disease modifying drugs. Non-steroidal anti-inflammatories block certain enzymes that increase inflammation in the joint but do nothing to alter the course of the disease. Corticosteroids are more powerful inflammation suppressors.

The third class, disease modifying drugs, are much more potent and have more concerning side effects but are also capable of slowing the progression of the disease. As I said earlier, none of these drugs were specifically designed for rheumatoid arthritis. For example, two common RA drugs are Plaquenil, an anti-malarial drug, and methotrexate, a drug used for cancer.

The good news is that our knowledge about the immune system has been growing by leaps and bounds and our exponential growth in knowledge won't be stopping anytime soon. The great news is that because of this new knowledge we now have drugs available to us that were developed specifically for rheumatoid arthritis. The word cure is finally being said.

Now let's take a deeper look into the immune system. The immune system is divided into three parts; physical barriers, which are the skin and mucus membranes, the innate, or nonspecific immune system, and the adaptive immune system.

Our physical barriers are our skin, which covers approximately 2 m² of surface area, and our mucus membranes encompassing approximately 400 m². Together they offer a considerable amount of protection, but invaders have had literally millions of years to develop strategies to infiltrate our barriers, which is why we have the other two parts of the immune system.

Our innate immune system is our second line of defense. Over 99% of animals get along fine carrying only the innate immune system and physical barriers. The innate immune system has evolved to detect and destroy common pathogens such as bacteria, virus, and parasites and plays a key role in the development and continuation of inflammation.

The adaptive immune system is the most complex and is only found in vertebrates. It is slower to act, but is also a lot more precise. It is in this part of the immune system that specific antibodies are made, and as I said earlier, cells of the adaptive immune system can recognize almost any organic molecule that exists.[14] Both the adaptive and innate immune systems are constantly in communication with each other and both play a vital part in the inflammatory process.[2]

This complex and intelligent army serves to keep us healthy and strong and it is helped in this process by other important systems. The immune, nervous, and endocrine systems communicate closely and interlink.

One example of the way in which the nervous system can become involved is that during acute inflammation the brain creates changes in behavior, inducing feelings of weakness, inability to concentrate, and depression. Interestingly, these are also symptoms of rheumatoid arthritis.

The endocrine system, consisting of glands which release hormones, is intricately involved with the whole process of inflammation and immunity as well, although the specifics of this are still largely unknown. What is known is that females have a two-to-tenfold higher incidence of autoimmune disease.

Now you can see quite clearly how the human body is made up of a lot more than just the sum of its parts. Each system is only the beginning of the story, and what really counts is how each part interacts with the other parts. Given the complexity of each system it's also quite clear why the majority of medical research focuses on each part separately. But to completely begin to heal your body it is imperative to look at the big picture. In medicine, this means looking beyond just symptom relief and I'm happy to report that a lot of doctors and researchers are doing just that.

So, let's begin with theories that are currently being considered.

---

[2] At the end of this chapter you'll find a description of the key players in the immune system and what is known about their role in rheumatoid arthritis, for those of you who are interested.

## It's In The Genes

In order for the immune system to operate effectively it has to be able to distinguish self from non-self. One way it does this is through a gene called HLA, or human leukocyte antigen. We all have a specific type of HLA that each of our cells display on its surface so that other cells can recognize it. People who carry a specific type of HLA, called HLA-DR4, are six times more likely to develop RA and twenty times more likely to develop juvenile diabetes.[15] What is a possible reason for this?

## Infection

Molecular mimicry. Sounds a bit underhanded and it is. We may have the advantage of spines, opposable thumbs, and big brains, but one celled organisms like bacteria and viruses have the advantage of billions of years of time to evolve. And in that time they have developed some tricky ways of evading their hosts. One particularly tricky way is to try to look like the self and they do this by coating themselves with amino acids very similar to the ones that our own cells have on their surface.

When a microbe is able to do this they confuse two cells of the adaptive immune system, B and T cells, into cross reacting with our own cells. One possible culprit in rheumatoid arthritis is mycobacterium tuberculosis which, when injected into rodents, will cause joint inflammation. This mycobacterium closely resembles the core structure of cartilage[16] Another interesting finding is that people with rheumatoid arthritis have almost ten times the amount of Epstein Barr virus, the virus commonly known as mono, in their blood.[17] There are many more infectious organisms that have or are being looked at as possible causes of autoimmune reactivity. It may turn out that more than one organism can end up causing RA in susceptible people. The confusion in our immune system happens when the invader carries receptors that look similar to our HLA gene receptor and there is probably more than one way that this can happen.

## *Self-Reactivity*

Another way self reactivity can happen is if immature B cells create autoantibodies, or antibodies to antibodies. Because the antibodies that B cells make are chosen in a completely random fashion and because one billion of them are made every day, the chances are pretty good that eventually this will happen and it does regularly, more and more the older we get. In rheumatoid arthritis the IgG anti-IgG autoantibody is formed and becomes extremely dangerous because it is small enough to leave the bloodstream and reach the joint. Once it gets there it can fool T cells into thinking there is an invader that needs to be attacked. This becomes a vicious cycle because these autoantibodies penetrate the joint lining and self perpetuate.[18]

The immune system learns to tolerate itself by getting rid of immature B and T cells that react to the tissue where they are born. If an immature T cell starts reacting to the cells in the thymus gland it will be killed off. This is an effective system but the question of how the body recognizes and gets rid of adult T and B cells that are reacting to the self is still a mystery that has yet to be solved.

Regulatory T cells may be a key to this mystery. Study of the role of regulatory T cells, also known as suppressor T cells, is still in its infancy as this type of T cell was only recently discovered. Because they suppress the response of the immune system however, they may prove to play a key role in autoimmune diseases like rheumatoid arthritis. The possibilities of defective regulatory T cells as a potential cause, and decreasing numbers of these cells in people with RA are both being looked at.[19]

## *Allergies*

There is an inverse correlation between susceptibility to traditional allergies and the likelihood of developing RA. People who are free from traditional allergies are actually more likely to develop RA. Interestingly though, the relationship between RA and food allergies is a subject that has seen a lot of conjecture and some research, personal testimonials, and strong opinions. Studies have shown certain dietary changes can benefit people with arthritis. A very low-fat diet showed improvements in one study while another demonstrated improvements in people following vegetarian diets. Most people have heard of the nightshade diet, which avoids potatoes, peppers, eggplants, and tomatoes. And then there is the gluten-free diet, which has worked wonders for some people. While these empirical results are intriguing, there hasn't been much research into why these diets work. Recently though, a study out of the University of Oslo in Norway found that the intestinal fluid of people with rheumatoid arthritis had higher level of antibodies to certain foods, including hen's eggs, cow's milk, pork, codfish, and cereal.[20] This supports the theory that food allergies contribute to joint inflammation.

A large percentage of the immune system is found in the gut, some say up to eighty percent. This is most likely because there is a large amount of potentially harmful material that comes through this area throughout day. The walls of the intestine are lined with tightly formed epithelial cells that keep food in the digestive tract and potential allergens out of the bloodstream. If the intestinal walls become more permeable this will allow molds, viruses, parasites, and food proteins to leak out.[21] Immune system activation from reactions to particles in the gut have been implicated in AIDS and diabetes and it wouldn't be a stretch to think that this could be an issue in rheumatoid arthritis.

## *Environmental Triggers*

If food allergies can activate the immune system it's possible that synthetic chemicals can do the same. There is a lot more research to be done in this area. One book, *Rheumatoid Arthritis: The Infection Connection,* was written by a researcher who developed severe rheumatoid arthritis and was able to improve dramatically through eliminating her exposure to environmental and food triggers. She discusses how microbes can cause, and food/chemical allergies can worsen arthritis and provides a comprehensive program to improve this situation.

## Stress

I talked earlier about how stress can lead to increased inflammation which ideally is stopped by the body once the stress is over. I also mentioned that stress creates inflammation because our bodies are designed for a world that no longer exists, a world that we lived in thousands of years ago. As far as we can tell now the stressors back then were a lot different and a stressful event was more likely to be one that involved physical injury. Turning on inflammation quickly made sense in situations like this. Before modern medicine the body had to be very effective at containing infections and inflammation was the most effective mechanism to do just that. In today's world stressors are much different. The stressors we experience often end up confusing the immune system and detrimental inflammation is more likely to result.

Compounding the problem, the adrenal glands of people with rheumatoid arthritis have a dampened response to stress. Lower levels of cortisol are produced leaving the body unable to turn off the inflammatory response even after the stressor is removed. This is called a dysregulation of the hypothalamic pituitary adrenal, or HPA axis. Women who have recently been through high levels of stress and recent use of contraceptive pills are more likely to develop autoimmune disease. Chronic stress can also predispose someone to an altered stress response[22]

Regardless of its role in the onset of RA, stress is a critical aspect of living well with the disease. None of us are immune to stress so learning how to deal with it well may mean the difference between a severe or minor flare up of your symptoms.

## Winning the Reverse Lottery

Obviously there is a lot that isn't known about rheumatoid arthritis and other autoimmune diseases. What is known however, is that it takes more than one event to create autoimmune disease; it's not easy to do. Winning the RA reverse lottery is just bad luck. The combination could look something like this: self reactive T and or B cells escape the bodies control systems and circulate through the bloodstream.  An individual undergoes stress, which lowers their immunity and allows an opportunistic infection to enter the body. This infectious agent happens to be able to mimic the body's own joint tissues. The self reactive cells now are stimulated to respond and this ends up creating a self perpetuating inflammatory response. Finally, an individual's genetic makeup can increase the probability that autoimmunity will happen when any of these circumstances emerge.

## *Strategies for Treatment*

As theories about the cause of rheumatoid arthritis are continuing to emerge, the way doctors are treating it is changing. Years ago, doctors were much more conservative in their initial approach and would only bring out the big guns if and when the arthritis became uncontrollable. This is called the pyramidal approach and the rationale for using it is to avoid the toxic side effects of the more potent drugs. Under the pyramidal approach non steroidal anti inflammatories are used and if they aren't effective after a few months gradually stronger drugs are introduced, one at a time, until the disease is under control. This can end up taking take years. The downside to this approach is that it doesn't prevent the joint destruction that can occur and isn't very effective at producing remission.

The inverted pyramid approach starts using stronger drugs immediately with or without non steroidal anti inflammatories. Within this approach are people who will combine two or more drugs at a time (combination therapy) and those that will only use one (monotherapy). The research is now showing that the inverted pyramid approach works much better at controlling early RA and that combination therapy works better than monotherapy. Fighting fire with fire seems to really work. Regardless of what caused the arthritis to start initially, turning down the viscous cycle of inflammation as quickly as possible makes a lot of sense.

While the future promises many more options for treatment, a possible arthritis vaccine and more individualized treatments, for now we are looking at four classes of drugs to choose from.

Let's look more closely at them:

## Non-Steroidal Anti-Inflammatory Drugs:

Include but are not limited to:

Relafen, Aspirin, Amigesic, Dolobid, Motrin, Advil, Orudis, Voltaren, Indocin, Clinoril, Tolectin, Lodine, Toradol, Feldene, Daypro, Aleve, Naprosyn

These drugs block the enzymes (Cox) that produce prostaglandins which are chemicals that increase inflammation. NSAIDS are some of the most commonly used drugs in the US. The medicines in this class work to alleviate the symptoms of joint pain and inflammation associated with arthritis but don't do anything to affect the course of the disease. They have been used so much that potential side effects are widely known. The most common is gastrointestinal toxicity because cox enzymes also protect the lining of the stomach. In fact it has been estimated that one-third of the cost of arthritis management is related to treating the adverse effects of NSAIDS. One subclass of NSAIDS, including Celebrex and Betra block only one cox enzyme, cox2, and because they are more selective there are less side effects in the gastrointestinal tract. One infamous cox 2 inhibitor, Vioxx, was withdrawn from the market because of its association with cardiac damage. The severity and high profile nature of Vioxx's adverse events have made people leery about using cox2 drugs. Given all of this information, the latest approach with using NSAIDS is to use a smaller doses, trying cox2 inhibitors with people who are at risk for gastrointestinal side effects, and to use another kind of drug, called a proton pump inhibitor, which will counteract side effects in the gastrointestinal tract.

## Corticosteroids

Including prednisone, Methylprednisone, Prednisolone, Betamethasone, Hydrocortisone, Dexamethasone

This class of drugs has a wide range of anti inflammatory effects. They are fast acting and powerful which make them great for severe, acute flare ups and bridge drugs to keep inflammation down for the time it takes for disease modifying drugs to start working. They can also be used in low doses for years and are often used in combination with disease modifying drugs. When steroids were first introduced in the 1940's they were thought to be a miraculous cure for arthritis because their effects were so dramatic. Before long doctors were prescribing very high doses to their patients and it was soon realized that the dramatic benefits of steroids were matched by equally dramatic side effects including insomnia, weight gain, fluid retention, osteoporosis, cataracts, hypertension, susceptibility to infection, excess hair growth, and muscle wasting. Steroids are a synthetic form of cortisol, which is produced naturally by the adrenal glands in our bodies, about 20 mg per day, in response to stress. Prednisone is four to five times more potent than cortisol and long term use will suppress the release of cortisol from the adrenals. Therefore, it is important to slowly wean off of them because it can take up to a year for adrenal function to return to normal. Because of their serious side effects steroids are always used with caution but when used appropriately they can be of great benefit.[23]

## Disease Modifying Anti-Rheumatic Drugs

This class of drugs is made up of a number of drugs most of which were initially used for other diseases but were found to have some benefit for RA. They have very little in common except for the fact that they can slow the progression of the disease.

*Methotrexate* for years has been the most frequently used and most effective DMARD. It was developed as a folic acid inhibitor in the 1940's. Methotrexate suppresses the immune system by diminishing T cells and cytokines. It also increases the release into the bloodstream of something called adenosine, a molecule widely found in the body that has many anti-inflammatory effects. Ingestion of caffeine can decrease the effectiveness of methotrexate. Including folic acid supplements will decrease side effects but won't decrease the anti inflammatory effects of the drug. [24]

Other widespread immune suppressant drugs include *Arava*, *Cyclosporine, D - penacillamine,* Cytoxan, Leukeran,and Imuran. These drugs all have some very toxic potential side effects because they are interfering not only with the inflammation of arthritis, but also suppressing the immune system cells that are vital to fighting infections. Liver and kidney damage are definite concerns for people taking these drugs as are increased susceptibility to infection and a possible increased risk of cancer. This is why doctors will monitor people taking these drugs much more closely.

*Tetracycline* and *Minocine*, Doxyclycline, and Clindomycine, are all antibiotics that are used by some rheumatologists. The use of these drugs is based on the theory that the cause of arthritis is a mycobacterium and was pioneered by a rheumatologist named Thomas McPherson Brown over fifty years ago. There are a few rheumatologists in this country who specialize in the antibiotic approach. Most rheumatologists, however, point out that improvements experienced from these drugs may be due to their anti-inflammatory effect and not their effect on mycobacterium. A great website to refer to for more information is www.rheumatic.org. There you will find research articles, protocols used by the doctors who specialize in this area, as well as support groups and frequently asked questions.

*Plaquenil* and *Flagelle* are anti-malarial drugs that are long standing DMARD's. The side effect profile for these drugs isn't as scary as immune suppressors, but neither are they as effective or fast acting as other DMARDS.

*Azulfidine* and *Gold* are both drugs that have been used for decades in the treatment of RA. Azulfidine is tolerated a lot better; in fact, injectable Gold is the most toxic of all the DMARD's used in the early stages of treatment. Up to 43%of people will stop taking it before positive gains are experienced. [25]

The problem with most DMARDs is that they tend to lose effectiveness over time and all have significant side effects which cause many people to stop using them. However, there are a lot to choose from and when used with care they can induce dramatic improvements for people with RA.

## Biologics

These are the newest drugs on the market. They were developed specifically for the treatment of rheumatoid arthritis and all have shown promising results. According to the National Cancer Institute, biologic drugs are "A substance that is made from a living organism or its products, and is used in the prevention, diagnosis, or treatment of cancer and other diseases. Biologic drugs include antibodies, interleukins, and vaccines."

Most biologics used in rheumatoid arthritis are aimed at one of three targets; cytokines, including interleuken 1 and tumor necrosis factor, T cells, and activated B cells. Some biologics are cultivated purely from human sources (Enbrel, Humira) and others use proteins from mice (Remicaide, Rituxan).

The biologics that target tumor necrosis factor were introduced first. TNF is one of the primary cytokines associated with inflammation and is found in very high numbers in inflamed joints.  The three TNF inhibitors currently used to treat RA include *Enbrel, Humira,* and *Remicaide.*

Interleukin 1 is another cytokine that promotes inflammation in the joint. *Kineret* is an approved drug that blocks IL-1.

*Orencia* decreases inflammation by blocking the activation of T cells.

B cell activation may be an important contributor to RA joint inflammation. The biologic drug *Rituxan* decreases the numbers of activated B cells which could cut off the inflammation at its source. [26]

Biologics have produced some dramatic results and even remissions in significant numbers of people. There are more biologics becoming available making this an exciting time for people with RA. The major side effects include infusion reactions and infections which can be severe enough to stop these treatments.

## *Enough Facts, Bring Out the Soapbox*

After a lifetime of being a patient and having personally experienced many of the treatments I've talked about in this chapter, I can't help but interject my own opinions. They are still my opinions- so take this next section with a grain of salt.

I think:

1.  Rheumatoid arthritis is more than one disease, more than one thing can cause it, and it takes a combination of things happening simultaneously in your body for it to erupt.
2.  Stress does exacerbate rheumatoid arthritis. Learning how to handle stress well is vital in living well with rheumatoid arthritis.
3.  Eventually, as different causes of RA are discovered, treatment will become individualized to meet the specific needs of each RA patient.
4.  An aggressive treatment approach early in the disease and during acute flare ups is a good idea. An aggressive approach over the long term is a bad idea and will do the body more harm than good.
5.  Researchers need to talk to each other more. Collaboration will be the key to fully understanding this complex disease.
6.  More research needs to be done in the areas of how food allergies and chemical toxins contribute to autoimmune disease. It just makes sense that the more your body is bombarded with foreign substances, the more likely the immune system will get overwhelmed and confused.
7.  Along those lines, all new chemicals need to be evaluated for toxicity the way that drugs are and the cumulative effects of exposure to multiple chemicals needs to be considered.

You may feel bombarded by now and you may also feel a bit overwhelmed.  With all of the questions out there and all of the possibilities for the causes and treatment of RA, what do you really know, what should you do? As I said in the beginning of this chapter the information I've given you can be approached like a buffet. It's okay if you don't really want to know or care about what causes arthritis. It's also okay if you just want to go to the doctor and have them decide what course of action is best for you. It's okay if you decide to dissect every piece of information in this chapter to try to put together the course of events that led to arthritis in your body, and if you want to be the one to decide about every pill that enters your throat. The most important thing here is to feel good about what you decide. I've been on both ends of this spectrum at different times in my life and both of them worked for me. With all of the unknowns out there the one thing I know for sure is that the right answer is the one that you feel most comfortable with.

## Key Players in the Immune System

**COMPLEMENT** is composed of approximately twenty proteins produced mainly in the liver and is very abundant in blood vessels and tissues. These proteins worked to punch holes in the cell walls of invading microorganisms so that they can be cleaned up by other cells. *Complement is active in the joint during the early stages of rheumatoid arthritis.*

**NEUTROPHILS** make up approximately 70% of white blood cells. We produce approximately 100 billion of these each day in our bone marrow. They are very effective killers and once activated they leave the bloodstream and enter tissues, where they "eat" invaders. The important point about neutrophils is that they act a bit like sharks during a feeding frenzy once they are activated. They easily get carried away, produce a lot of free radicals, and damage normal tissues in the course of doing their job. *There are very few neutrophils in normal tissues but are abundant in the fluid of people with rheumatoid arthritis.*

Unlike neutrophils **MACROPHAGES** are long-lived, their life span can be years. A macrophage is a large cell that has many functions and it is responsible for initiating numerous defense strategies upon encountering a pathogen. Once they are activated macrophages begin to use one of over a hundred different substances they have at their disposal to constrict and dilate different blood vessels at the site, contributing to the swelling that is so common in the joints of people with rheumatoid arthritis. They also produce cytokines, hormone-like protein messengers that communicate and recruit other cells in the immune system to increase inflammation. For example, macrophages can release tumor necrosis factor, or TNF, which is frequently the first cytokine to be secreted during the inflammatory response. TNF triggers a cascade response which involves the secretion of other cytokines such as interleukins 1, 6, and 8. A macrophage is never lazy. When it isn't stomping out invaders it works as a garbage collector in the body, eating cellular debris. *While macrophages are found in large numbers in the*

135

*thickened synovial lining of people with RA, and also in the area of the joint lining that blood vessels are located, the role macrophages play in RA is not understood at this time. One theory is that macrophages may enter a self-perpetuating cycle once inflammation is initiated. By releasing cytokines, macrophages activate other cells such as* **fibroblasts** *(cells that make up connective tissue,) which elicit the pro-inflammatory response of cells like* **prostaglandins** *and* **neutrophils**. *Completing the cycle, this response ends up re-activating the macrophages.*

Confused yet? And we're not even done! Now, like me, you can fully appreciate why medical researchers have their work cut out for them.

**FIBROBLASTS** are cells that provide the structural framework for connective tissue and collagen. They are involved in wound healing and inflammation. *Along with macrophages, large numbers of fibroblasts are found in the synovial lining of the RA affected joint. And like macrophages they can secrete large amounts of cytokines as well as prostaglandins and enzymes that erode bone and cartilage. Tissue damage stimulates the production of more fibroblasts, beginning yet another vicious cycle of inflammation and tissue damage.*

**PROSTAGLANDINS** are derived from fatty acids and are technically hormones They have many functions but the important one with regard to RA is that *they can promote inflammation once they are synthesized in the joint. Anti-inflammatory drugs and steroid drugs both decrease prostaglandin synthesis.*[27]

**CYTOKINES** are messenger molecules similar to hormones that are used by the cells of the immune system to control the response of other molecules. *A number of cytokines are found in the joints of people with rheumatoid arthritis, including interleukin 1, 6, and 8 and tumor necrosis factor (TNF). A few of the new biologic drugs specifically target these cytokines.*[28]

**MAST CELLS** are part of the innate immune system. These cells are very long lived and can survive for years in tissues. When activated, they release granules which recruit different types of white blood cells including B and T cells , neutrophils, natural killer cells, and macrophages. Mast cells also release large amounts of the cytokine tumor necrosis factor, and histamine which increases the permeability of blood vessels. *In the joints of people with RA mast cells are found in the layer of tissue containing blood vessels. Normally, this area has very few cells. Some research into rheumatoid arthritis has focused on mast cells which may be the driving force behind sustained joint inflammation.*

**LYMPHOCYTES** are comprised of T cells and B cells.  Lymphocytes are the key players of the adaptive immune system and also most likely the key to how autoimmune diseases like rheumatoid arthritis develop and persist.

**T CELLS** are created in the bone marrow and mature in the thymus gland. We have about a trillion of them in our body. T cells can recognize when cells have become infected by an invader. There are three kinds of T cells.  Killer T cells directly attack infected cells.  Helper T cells recognize antigens on the surface of cells and can either stimulate B cells and other cells to attack the antigen or produce cytokines. Regulatory T cells have an extremely important role in the immune system, helping to distinguish cells that are part of the self and those that are foreign, and in controlling the response of other T cells. There is much that still isn't known about these important cells. What is known is that if they aren't functioning correctly autoimmune disease will often result. *Helper T cells become overactive in rheumatoid arthritis and stimulate cells to produce autoantibodies which are directed at the body's own cells.  This autoantibody is derived from IGg, one of five types of antibodies.  The IGg antibody sticks to organisms and enhances cell destruction by neutrophils and macrophages.*

**B CELLS** are created in the bone marrow at a rate of approximately one billion per day. On the surface of every B cell is a unique receptor that recognizes a specific antigen, or foreign substance. The fact that each B cell has a unique receptor and that they are so abundant is the reason that they are able to recognize almost any organic molecule in the world. Once a B cell recognizes an antigen it creates antibodies against that substance. It will also replicate, creating clones that will quickly eliminate the foreign body. If a B cell is activated once it will create a memory of the experience so that the next time it recognizes it's antigen it will activate antibody production a lot quicker. *In rheumatoid arthritis there are antibodies created against the IgG antibody, called the rheumatoid factor. There are also IgM antibodies that have attached to the tails of IgG antibodies. These are called autoantibodies because they are antibodies to the self which creates an autoimmune situation. Self-reactive B cells are being investigated as possible causes of rheumatoid arthritis.[29]*

# *Chapter Four Worksheet*

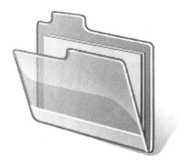

- What Do I Want to Learn More About

# WHAT DO I WANT TO LEARN MORE ABOUT?

My immune system?

_____
_____
_____
_____
_____
_____

Arthritis drug options?

_____
_____
_____
_____
_____
_____

My family history?

_____
_____
_____
_____
_____
_____

Strategies for treatment?

_____
_____
_____
_____
_____
_____

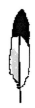

*I was in a tea shop the other day writing this book when I couldn't help but overhear a conversation between a young man in his early twenties and a young woman who couldn't have been a day over nineteen. He was mentoring her on how to sell a nutritional drink called Xango, which is made out of a highly nutritious fruit from Asia called the mangosteen. I know this because I've taken it before and I also know about the concept of network marketing because I've been a member of a supplement company myself. Despite trying to block them out, I kept hearing snippets of the conversation and the more I heard, the more dismayed I became. The man said things like "Don't go after your uncle who sits on the couch every day watching television, go to natural food stores and find people who are already interested in their health." "The people you really want to go after are the people who already have a disease. These are the people who are going to be most interested in what you have to say because they already have an incentive. These are the people you are going to make money from."*

*Actually, there is nothing inherently wrong with any of the things this young guy was saying. He's right. The reason I became so upset by him was that I could imagine these words being exchanged by thousands and thousands of people every day who are trying to cash in on the new wellness industry and also by the professionals working for huge companies that spend trillions of dollars every year marketing their drugs to people like us and our doctors.  Xango and the many other supplements out there may be very good, but how can I really trust someone whose true motivation is to make a buck? How do I handle being a target of these people and still take care of my body's needs? How do I decipher hype from fact?*

*This has been an ongoing quandary for me for many years, and in the process I've learned quite a lot. I've learned how to alter my diet to discourage inflammation and I've learned that there are many great supplements available that have really made a positive difference in my life. I've also learned that what works for my body can be very different from what will help someone else, that too much of a good thing is bad, and that my own body's needs are constantly changing.*

*I've often become overwhelmed in the process. Finding the right balance of eating in a healthy manner and placating people around me who are entrenched in their own views and attitudes about food. Believing in many a supplement only to be disappointed with quite a few.*

*I now know that a healthy dose of skepticism is a good thing when approaching claims of anti-inflammatory remedies, that trust should be doled out like a pauper and fortitude should be held onto like a king. I know that my diet is one thing I have control over and as long as I don't use this control to fill an emotional need, I can use it to help myself be healthy despite my diagnosis of RA.*

# Chapter Five:

## Nutrition, Are You What You Eat?

"He that takes medicine and neglects diet,
wastes the skill of the physician."
                            - *Chinese Proverb*

Food is many things and satisfies us on many levels. Food is delicious, comforting, functional, culturally relative, and can inspire awe, fear, guilt, and pleasure, sometimes all at the same time. Food can be associated with fat or starvation; it all depends on where you are and when you've last eaten. Food is a necessity for life and health and has never been more of a minefield in this country. Compare Americans with people in other cultures and you'll become acutely aware of how differently we approach food. We've lost much of the reverence, enjoyment, and social time that is a natural accompaniment to food in most other places. We've replaced this with convenience, apprehension, and isolation.

Food is tied to how we feel about ourselves emotionally, hence the term emotional eating. Many people spend a lot of time altering their food content to make themselves feel and look better and a lot of money on diets and supplements that may or may not work. The percentage of women in this country who say they have an eating disorder of some kind is an astounding sixty-five percent. Food is tied to body image, self esteem, and self control. This era of improved nutritional knowledge has succeeded in muddying the waters even more.

The food industry has molded what we eat and the way we eat it; some food is trendy and other food is ignored. Although the variety of food we have access to in this country is unprecedented, the variety of food we actually eat is dismal.

Food isn't as simple as it looks and we all need to acknowledge that when we begin the process of investigating food and health. Although there are definite links to food consumption and health (look into the Mediterranean diet) as well as food consumption and ill health (check out the movie Super Size Me), there is no definitive answer about who should eat what.

Changing the way you eat isn't as simple as it seems either because first you have to change your habits, deal with your emotions around the decision, and most disturbingly, deal with the emotional reactions of everyone around you. Changing your eating habits can invite ridicule (ask any vegetarian), unsolicited commentary and advice, or apprehension among the people you surround yourself with. Most people are acutely aware of some things in their ordinary diet they should cut out but would be surprised at other dietary changes they never thought of. Most people don't know who to believe. Most people would do well to believe very little of what they hear and to try to understand what works best for their body by doing a bit of research on their own.

## *Wading through the Hype*

Wading through all the hype has led me to three conclusions that I think every person with rheumatoid arthritis can work with:

- Food can be used to help influence your tendency towards inflammation.

- Chronic inflammation creates a need in the body for extra nutrition.

- Medications used for arthritis can deplete certain nutrients that are necessary for health.

Let's talk more about this.

In an ideal world your diet would provide you with all of the nutrition that you need. Unfortunately, in today's world it takes knowledge and work to do this. So, what is wrong with our food options today and how does this relate to arthritis?

The first challenge we face is that our soil has been depleted, a fact that has been proven more than once in studies both in the US and in England. One dramatic demonstration of this was shown in a study at the University of Texas, Austin's Biochemical Institute. Looking at USDA data on the nutritional content of forty-three fruits and vegetables, six out of thirteen nutrients that were looked at were found to have declined significantly including riboflavin (38 %), vitamin C (15%), and protein (6%).As a result we have to eat a lot more to get what we need. I've noticed that recently the recommended daily intake of fruits and vegetables keeps going up. It used to be 5-8, now it's up to 9-12. That's a lot of chewing!

Secondly, we are buying food that travels a long way to get to our table which means it is green harvested. Food that isn't vine ripened is a lot less nutritious; it's the last 24 hours when the majority of phytonutrients, so important for health, are manufactured in the plant. The jury is still out on genetically modified food, however it is important to know that sixty to seventy percent of the processed food we eat contains genetically modified ingredients. The most commonly modified crops are soybeans, corn, cotton, and rapeseed oil. This means that when you eat foods with high fructose corn syrup, canola or cottonseed oil, or soybean you can assume that they were genetically modified unless they are labeled otherwise.[30] The important thing to remember is that the more you modify something the more likely it is that the immune system will get confused and not recognize it as food. As a person who has a predisposition to an immune system that goes into overdrive, I want to make darn sure that I don't provoke it. On the contrary, I want to decrease the inflammatory load as much as I possibly can.

Which brings me to all those chemicals that get put in and on our food for various reasons. One scary statistic is that there have been over 75,000 new chemicals introduced since 1930. Only about 7% have been tested on adults and 3% on children for safety. In 2003, the Environmental Working Group concluded the first study that thoroughly analyzed the amounts of chemicals in humans. They found the presence of, on average, 91 chemicals in the people tested.[31]

I always thought it was odd that the government tests chemicals for human safety in isolation. It's not as if we are only exposed to one at a time. What happens with the cumulative effect of the hormones and antibiotics we're getting in our milk, the pesticides on our grapes, the genetically modified tomato? I think I know one likely possibility since every chronic disease category is going up in this country. Cancer, diabetes, heart disease are all skyrocketing despite some wonderful medical advances. What science and medicine are doing in response to theses crises are more treatments, medicines, tests, DNA screens. That's great, but not enough. What we need to do is to take the initiative, go back to basics, be aware of the environmental challenges we face in our daily life, and do everything we possibly can to decrease the amount of toxins we take into our bodies. Less toxic stress means less inflammatory load.

**Let's break this down a bit more and look at what we are dealing with.**

A. Depleted, green harvested food source resulting in less vitamins, minerals, phytochemicals in our diet

B. Toxins in our water, food, air

C. A standard American diet that is highly processed, heavy on animal products, and emphasizes only a few foods

D. A body that has the tendency to be in a chronically inflamed state

E. Ingestion of drugs that may deplete certain vitamins and minerals

F. Ingestion of drugs that may impair our digestive function

What do we do with this information? Is it time to throw in the towel and start eating ice cream? I've decided to wait until I'm 90 to do this, I figure if I've lived that long I deserve to eat ice cream for breakfast, lunch, dinner, and even a midnight snack if I want. Until then I have another plan.

Arthritis creates inflammation; inflammation creates free radicals, or pro oxidants. These unstable molecules lack an electron and are constantly seeking out other molecules to steal electrons from so that they can become stable. This creates a problem because the molecule they steal from is now a free radical which creates a vicious cycle and ends up contributing to disease unless there are plenty of antioxidants to deal with them. Therefore, a person with arthritis needs plenty of antioxidants at hand. Where does one find these helpful substances?

## *Food is Good*

In the rainbow colors of fresh fruits and vegetables. The recommendation of nine to twelve servings of fruits and vegetables every day is for a healthy individual with no health challenges. A person with arthritis needs to eat smart and possibly supplement his/her diet with quality antioxidants. Eating smart means to make all those fruits and vegetables count and that's where organic, in season, local, farm fresh foods can help. As I said earlier, the apples you get in the grocery store in the winter were green harvested and most likely have been sitting in storage for months. To get the freshest food possible eat foods that are in season. How do you know what foods are in season when? These days you can get most anything you'd want at anytime you want. The best way to shop in season is to shop locally. Make a habit of going to your farmer's market if there is one near you, and if not look into co-ops. Co-ops will often deliver right to your door, for a price.

**Whenever possible eat organic food.** Organic food is a perfect example of the saying "You get what you pay for." On average organic produce has 30% higher levels of antioxidants, 21% more iron, 27% more vitamin C, 29.3% more magnesium, and 13.6% more phosphorus.[32]This is obviously quite a difference and the benefits you'll get by eating more organic food will quickly add up.

**Have fun with your food**. We are all creatures of habit and that goes for how we eat as well. Getting stuck in a food rut is easy to do, I can be as guilty as anyone. For our bodies though, this may have the consequences of having to process a lot of one thing, and try to make do without something else that may be extremely important in keeping us functioning well. Can you guess what the top two fruits consumed by Americans are? (Bananas and apples)[33]The top five vegetables (Iceberg lettuce, french fries, potatoes, potato chips, and canned tomatoes )[34] The top two grains? (Wheat and corn) What percentage of your diet contains these common foods? When was the last time you ate a turnip? A sweet potato? Kale? How many people know what a turnip is let alone have ever eaten one?

My point is that even people who think they eat a healthy diet are misinforming themselves if they don't eat a variety of foods. Dr. Andrew Weil, an expert on nutrition and health as well as an author of numerous books on the subject, talks about eating foods of all colors. And he isn't talking about the colors you find in a bag of M&M's! He means that if you eat fruits and vegetables containing greens, reds, oranges, purples, and yellows throughout the day and the week you will be ensuring that your body is getting all the phytonutrients it needs to maintain and improve health. Phytonutrients are compounds that actually give fruits and vegetables their color and have numerous health promoting benefits including modulating the immune system, providing antioxidants, protecting against cancer and decreasing inflammation. What would this look like? Zucchini, lettuce, tomato, cherry, sweet potato, mango, eggplant, blackberry, banana, parsnip, that about covers it for a few days.

The way that I've made this fun is to buy one new item in the produce section that I haven't tried each time I go shopping and then figure out what to do with it. In this way I've discovered a bunch of new favorite foods: beets, parsnips, rutabaga, dates, portabella mushrooms. I can whip up a dish with any of those and satisfy most palates. I try this with grains as well, and am constantly amazed at how uncreative the food industry is. Millet, quinoa, amaranth, spelt, these are all really good and not at all hard to cook with. Even picky eaters will be surprised and really picky eaters can be tricked. All you have to do is substitute spelt for wheat, or barley flakes for oats in cookie recipes and nobody will be the wiser.

Dr. Weil also talks about using an anti-inflammatory diet as a way to decrease your tendency towards inflammation. The way you eat can create a pro-inflammatory state or an anti-inflammatory state. Eating to decrease your inflammatory load will help not only arthritis, but also your tendency toward other inflammatory conditions like heart disease and diabetes. The way to do this is to consider both the kinds of macronutrients you eat, which include fats, proteins, and carbohydrates, as well as the micronutrients, including vitamins, minerals, and the phytonutrients I just talked about.

**Let's start with fats.** Fats get a bad rap, I wonder if it's because of their name. Imagine being named fat, especially in this country where being fat means discrimination and judgment. So, once you can get beyond the name remember that fats are vital to the health of our skin, nervous system, and eating the right kinds of fats can actually help you build lean muscle. Fatty acids are incorporated into all of our cell membranes so when it comes to fats you really are what you eat. Most importantly though, the body needs fatty acids to synthesize hormones and other substances that either increase or decrease inflammation.

There are four kinds of fats. Saturated fat is the fat you get from animal sources and some plant oils like coconut, and contributes to increasing inflammation. As someone with RA it is important to limit consumption of saturated fats.[35]

Trans fats are by many accounts one of the worst foods you can eat, and include margarine, vegetable shortening, and partially hydrogenated vegetable oils. The process of turning liquid oils into solids involves altering them chemically.

Like many advances of the modern world that have ended up being trouble (think plastics, pesticides, and many would say, cell phones!), partial hydrogenation was invented with the best of intentions in mind.

Before partial hydrogenation people cooked with lard and butter which were eventually linked to heart disease and high cholesterol. As a way to solve this health problem manufacturers wanted to use plant oils, but because these oils are unstable when exposed to heat they used the process of hydrogenation.[36] By adding a hydrogen atom the new partially hydrogenated fats had a higher melting point and a longer shelf life. Crisco was the first trans fat on the market and appeared in 1911. As the health consequences of saturated fats became more widely known, and manufacturers were able to use partial hydrogenation with great results, this type of fat became widely used in most processed foods.

Trans fats are now known to directly increase inflammation, and they also increase levels of harmful cholesterol contributing to heart disease. In fact, trans fat increases the risk of heart disease more than any other macro nutrient and is responsible for eighty two deaths each day.[37] A minute amount of trans fats are found in some foods like peas, cabbage, cow, goat and sheep meats, cow's milk and pomegranates, but because they are naturally occurring and their amounts are so low they aren't a concern. The bottom line is to read labels and don't buy foods that list hydrogenated or partially hydrogenated oil as an ingredient.

The last two types of fats are monounsaturated and polyunsaturated fats. They are both healthy for us and essential nutrients which means we have to get them from our food; we can't manufacture them on our own. Polyunsaturated fats can be broken down into omega 3's and omega 6's. Omega 3's are needed to create anti-inflammatory materials and are found in oily fish, leafy greens, walnuts, flax seeds, hemp seeds, soy and canola oil, and sea vegetables among others. Omega 6's are needed as well, but in smaller amounts and they can potentially increase inflammation because one thing that they do is assist in manufacturing prostaglandins, chemicals that are directly responsible for increasing or decreasing inflammation. As a point of reference, anti inflammatories like aspirin work to decrease prostaglandin synthesis.

Unfortunately, the food we eat in our modern world is full of omega 6's and almost bereft of omega 3's. It is estimated that the modern diet consists of twenty times more omega 6's than omega 3's, while in the

Stone Age our consumption of these two was almost equal.[38] Virtually all of the snack foods we eat, as well as fast food, is packed with omega 6's and has none of the vital omega 3's. And we have passed this inequity in our diet onto our domesticated animals including cows, poultry, and even farm raised fish. This ends up directly affecting us because when we eat these animals, their meat is high in the omega 6's and low in omega 3's. In order to deal with this inequity it is really important to make a point of including omega 3 rich foods into your diet, and trying to reduce your consumption of snack foods that contain oils.

The other thing to keep in mind is that plant oils go rancid easily and that heating oils also changes them chemically, making them harmful. Some oils withstand heat better than others and those are the oils that you should cook with. The best thing to do is cook with as little oil as possible and consume your good oils at room temperature.

Here's a list of the good, bad, and ugly when it comes to oils:

| Good | Limit | Avoid |
|---|---|---|
| **Bake With:** | Regular Safflower Oil | Partially Hydrogenated Oils |
| Canola Oil | Regular Sunflower Oil | Hydrogenated Oils |
| High Oleic Safflower Oil | Corn Oil* | Margarine |
| **Stir Fry With:** | Cottonseed Oil* | Vegetable Shortening |
| Extra Virgin Olive Oil | Palm Kernel Oil | |
| Olive Oil | Peanut Oil | |
| **Use at Room Temp Only:** | Coconut Oil | |
| Flax Seed Oil | Butter | |
| Hemp Seed Butter and Oil | | |
| Cod Liver Oil/Fish Oil | | |
| Avocados and Oil | | |

*\* These oils are more likely to be genetically modified*

So, to sum up, eat more omega 3 rich foods, limit processed foods and saturated fats, use oil sparingly when cooking, and most of all, if you do nothing else, avoid trans fats.

Next let's talk about protein. Protein is extremely important for building lean muscle and repairing tissues. Protein won't directly affect inflammation either way, what influences your inflammatory load is what comes along with the protein you eat. This means that when it comes to protein you need to be concerned about the fat that it contains as well as the environmental toxins that the protein was exposed to. Animals are much higher up on the food chain than plants and will contain a lot more toxins in the form of pesticides, mercury, and anything else that the animal was exposed to during their life. Grass fed animals are always a better choice because they will have more omega 3 fatty acids. Animals that are grain fed will be much higher in omega 6's and arachidonic acid, which create inflammation. This is why poultry is not always the best choice when it comes to meat. Most poultry is grain fed, so when you eat chicken and turkey you will want to eat the white meat, or leaner part of the animal.

Surprisingly, when it comes to red meat, leaner is not always better. Once again, this is related to the ratio of omega 3's and 6's. Omega 3's may be found in the fatty portion and the 6's in the meatier portion, so if you only eat the lean cut you'll be losing out on your omega 3's.[39] However, all red meat will have saturated fat as well which is pro-inflammatory so a diet rich in red meat isn't a great idea. Eating fish may expose you to mercury but, eating some types of fish will also give you the vital omega 3's that your body needs and are some of the best anti-inflammatory foods you can eat. If mercury exposure concerns you the way to get around this is to eat fish that are smaller and emphasize fish that is rich in omega 3's. One thing to keep in mind though is that farm raised salmon is best avoided at all costs; it is the most inflammatory fish you can eat.[40] Once again, this is because they are fed a grain based diet. They are also pumped full of artificial food coloring once they are killed to make them appear pink just like their wild cousins.

There isn't any conclusive evidence that becoming a vegetarian will help arthritis but learning to incorporate vegetable sources of protein into your diet might be a good idea if you are concerned about decreasing your inflammatory load. Last but not least, low or no fat dairy is better than full fat because of the saturated fat it contains.

| Emphasize | Limit |
| --- | --- |
| Fatty, Cold Water Fish like Salmon, Tuna, Sardines, Sablefish, Char, and Mackerel | Farmed Salmon |
| | Organ Meats |
| Vegetable Protein | Poultry Dark Meat |
| Grass Fed Meat | High Fat Dairy |
| Low Fat Dairy | |

Finally, let's talk about carbohydrates. The issue with carbohydrates is elevated blood sugar. Increasing the amount of sugar in your blood results in something called glycation, a bodily process that can have numerous detrimental effects on health over time, including inflammation. The end products of glycation actually increase C reactive protein, a protein produced as part of the inflammatory process. The way you decrease spikes in blood sugar is to emphasize whole grains, avoid high fructose corn syrup, limit sugar, refined food and white flour, and eat some protein with your meal to slow down digestion. For those of you who want to investigate this in detail, you can look into the glycemic index and glycemic load, both measures of how quickly and strong blood sugar is elevated after eating a certain food.

| Emphasize | Limit | Avoid |
| --- | --- | --- |
| Whole Grains | Processed Foods | High Fructose Corn Syrup |
| Vegetables | White Flour | |

## *Eat to Erase Inflammation*

In the book *The Inflammation Free Diet Plan*, Julius Torelli, MD created and explains a system for ranking food according to their tendency to create inflammation. The book has a comprehensive list of common foods, and their inflammatory rating is sometimes surprising.

**Here I'm going to list a few of the highest anti-inflammatory foods on his list:**

| | |
|---|---|
| Anchovies | Cayenne Pepper |
| Cod Liver Oil | Halibut |
| Arctic Char | Carrot Juice |
| Collard Greens | Kale |
| Bass | Mackerel, Jack or Pacific |
| Curry Powder | Wild Salmon, Fresh or Canned |
| Blue Fin Tuna | Turmeric |
| Spinach | Ginger |

You may notice a few things from this list. Fish is a great addition to your diet, green is good (especially green vegetables), and certain spices can make a huge impact on whether a meal is anti-inflammatory. The key thing to remember is that for most people it won't take a huge dietary overhaul for the creation of real positive change in your diet. All that is necessary is the incorporation of a few key ingredients, maybe changing how you cook a bit, and eliminating a few bad guys from your dietary repertoire.

Using food as a way to treat and alleviate disease is something that is second nature for people in many cultures, especially in the East, but for some reason here in the West we have created a strange dichotomy between food and medicine. We have the saying, "You are what you eat," but we don't really take this seriously, and the term 'health nut" is used in a derogatory sense. The idea of using specific foods to alter specific disease states is now, thankfully, being more widely investigated and there is a whole field of nutrition called functional nutrition that uses this concept in its approach to health.

The anti-inflammatory foods I just listed would qualify as something called functional foods because they have the ability to create real change in the body just like anti-inflammatory medicines. Something to keep your eyes peeled for are new functional foods that are made specifically for decreasing inflammation. Researchers in food science are actually patenting ways to add edible seed oils and flours that are natural anti-inflammatories to common foods and food companies are using this new knowledge to create new products.[41] This is exciting research that has the potential to transform the food industry and the health of us consumers in hugely positive ways. As consumers, though, we do have to be aware of how this industry is regulated and how claims are made.

Now let's talk about some other functional foods or supplements that can be added to your diet. One type of functional food for arthritis is food that contains high levels of probiotics, or good bacteria, which line the intestines and help to limit inflammatory responses in the gut.[42] These foods include fermented vegetables and yogurt. Probiotic supplements are also available at any health food store. Since non-steroidal anti-inflammatories alter the balance of bacteria in the intestine and antibiotics wipe out bacteria altogether it's always important to take probiotics after a course of antibiotics and along with NSAIDS. Another reason that probiotics are so important is that they help you to assimilate and metabolize key nutrients. Realistically it's not what you eat that's most important, it's what you absorb, and probiotics will help you with this.

**Ginger** is another anti-inflammatory all star. It has been researched widely and found to decrease two pro-inflammatory immune cells, prostaglandins and leukotrines, which, by the way, is what anti-inflammatory drugs do. Ginger can decrease pain and swelling, and adverse reactions are extremely rare.[43] Ginger is used widely in Asia and also has antioxidant, anti-tumor, and anti-nausea benefits and is high in calcium.

**Turmeric** is a spice that you'll want to try if you have inflammation. It is the main ingredient in curry powder and is a member of the ginger family. Turmeric is a mild Cox 2 inhibitor but doesn't have the side effects of anti- inflammatory drugs. Animal studies have shown improvement in arthritis symptoms and turmeric may protect against cancer and Alzheimer's disease as well. Okinawans, one of the longest living populations on earth, regularly drink a cold turmeric tea.[44]

**Cayenne pepper** is a nutritional all-star and has been used medicinally for circulatory issues, pain, digestion, and heart health. It helps to rebuild tissues in the stomach and intestines and stimulates the production of hydrochloric acid in the stomach which is necessary for the digestion of proteins. It simulates peripheral circulation and organ secretions, helps with dyspepsia, normalizes blood pressure, and assists in lymphatic function.[45]

The question of whether to supplement your diet with vitamins and minerals is an ongoing one. Studies constantly contradict themselves. One study will extol the anti-inflammatory benefits of vitamin E, and the next will say it causes cancer. To me, this is another demonstration that you can prove just about anything you want. The reality beyond all the hype is that too much of even a good thing can be bad, vitamins are not meant to be taken in isolation, and a synthetic form of anything can be detrimental. Those of us who have taken medications which are synthetic forms of plants can attest to that. So, studies using vitamins or minerals may or may not use synthetic forms and the dosages that are taken will all be variable as well, hence the contradictory results. What we all need to realize is that ideally we need to ingest vital nutrients in the form of real food because the vitamins in food will be accompanied by other nutrients that enhance its absorption. However, as I stated earlier, our food isn't as nutrient dense as it used to be and our diet is higher in processed foods which are nutrient depleted, so supplementing with certain vital nutrients can be a really good idea if you have rheumatoid arthritis as long as you use food based supplements. If your supplement is food based the label will say so because the company making it will want you to know. The ideal situation to aim for is to incorporate powerhouse foods into your diet that are packed with antioxidants and nutritionally dense, rotate these foods so you aren't always eating one or two of them, and also supplement with a few well known anti- inflammatory nutrients as well.

Let's talk about powerhouse foods:

*Broccoli*: Has been called the number one anti-cancer vegetable, containing compounds which block cell mutations and block the growth of tumors. It is only twenty-four calories per cup raw, has two and a half times the RDA for vitamin C, is an excellent source of calcium, and is rich in carotene, vitamin K, and iron.

*Papaya*: The most nutrient dense of fruits, the papaya exceeds the RDA for vitamins A and C and is also rich in potassium and fiber. Try an easy papaya salad by mixing papaya, cilantro, lime juice, balsamic vinegar, extra virgin olive oil, and a bit of red onion. You can also add some avocado to make it extra nutritious.

*Sweet potatoes:* This delicious vegetable is rich in vitamin A. So rich that one cup of mashed sweet potato will give you eight times the recommended daily allowance of this vitamin. Sweet potatoes are also rich in protease inhibitors which protect against cancer and viruses. Dark orange vegetables like sweet potatoes, carrots, and winter squash all have been shown to protect against lung cancer.

*Kale*: Kale is a powerful cancer fighter, rich in carotenoids, vitamins A, C, riboflavin, niacin, calcium, magnesium, iron, sulphur, sodium, potassium, phosphorus, and chlorophyll. Eat kale both raw and cooked for the most nutritional benefit.

*Berries*: All berries supply fiber, and anthocyanins, plant pigments which convey anti-inflammatory, anti-carcinogenic, and antioxidant effects.

One stand out is cherries, which have been shown to improve arthritis symptoms.

*Parsley*: Adding a bit of parsley to your food will give you a huge nutritional boost. Parsley is high in vitamins A, B1, B- complex, C, potassium, manganese, phosphorus, calcium, and iron. Make hummus with garbanzo beans, lemon, garlic, cumin, red onion, tahini, and parsley or add parsley to soups.

*Carrots:* This crunchy treat reduces acidic conditions and benefits the skin, reducing inflammation in the mucus membranes. Carrots are rich in beta carotene, silicon (which aids calcium metabolism), potassium, soluble fiber, and contain vitamin C.

*Avocado*: Avocado is a fruit that is hearty and healthy enough to be a meal. It has protein, vitamins A, D, and E, 14 minerals including high amounts of copper and iron, phosphorus, magnesium, calcium, and more potassium than bananas.

*Asparagus*: Your kidneys and liver will thank you for eating this diuretic vegetable, as it stimulates the function of these two vital organs. Asparagus is rich in A, B- complex, and C, selenium, potassium, manganese, iron, asparagine, and rutin (good for your capillaries.)

*Peas:* The lowly pea, the very pea that we all were forced to eat as little kids, is another reminder that mother knows best. A 3/4 cup serving of peas have as much protein as an egg without the saturated fat and cholesterol and as much soluble fiber as kidney beans, helping to regulate blood sugar. Peas contain large amounts of vitamin A, vitamin C, phosphorus and have been shown to prevent appendicitis and ulcers, and lower blood pressure.[46]

*Spinach:* If it's good enough for Popeye.... Spinach is one of the top ten most nutritious vegetables. The high amount of chlorophyll and iron in spinach helps it to build and cleanse the blood. Its sulphur content helps the skin and hair. Spinach is also rich in vitamin C, folic acid, vitamin A, and calcium, although the calcium in spinach may be neutralized by its high oxalic content.

*Quinoa:* This ancient grain, the staple food for the Incas over 5000 years ago, is actually a seed related to the spinach family. Since it cooks and tastes like a grain it can easily replace cooked grains in most recipes. Quinoa is considered a super food with good reason. It is a complete protein, containing all nine essential amino acids, calcium, magnesium, manganese, iron, fiber, B vitamins, phosphorus, potassium, copper, and zinc. One cup of cooked quinoa has eleven grams of protein, more than a cup of milk. Not bad for a lowly "grain."

*Sea Vegetables:* Otherwise known as seaweeds, they are widely consumed in Japan and has been attributed to the low rates of cancer in this part of the world. Seaweeds are easier to add to the diet than most people think and there are many good reasons to make the effort. Seaweeds are a natural source of trace minerals, are rich in calcium, iodine, iron, potassium, phosphorus, manganese, sodium, zinc, vitamins A, C, and B complex, and contain protein and essential fatty acids. Seaweeds aid in endocrine gland function, especially the thyroid, reduce blood cholesterol, and improve the health of the nails, hair, bones, and teeth.[47] Nori rolls can be used as a wrap and filled with vegetables, rice, and avocado, kelp can be toasted and eaten like chips, the powdered form can be used as a flavoring, and kombu can be added to rice, beans, or soups as a flavor enhancer.

## Drugs and Nutrition

Who knew that drugs for arthritis deplete certain vitamins? I didn't until I started taking methotrexate and was told that I needed to take folic acid. Since then I've learned that many of the drugs commonly used for RA deplete some significant vitamins. Here's a list of some of these adapted from the book, *The Nutritional Cost of Drugs*, written by Ross Pelton and James LaVelle.

**Methotrexate**: Depletes *folic acid*, which can result in some serious health complications including anemia, birth defects, cervical dysplasia, nausea, insomnia, fatigue, depression, hair loss, weight loss, headache, and increase your risk for infections, cancer, and heart disease.

**Corticosteroids**: Long term use of these drugs results in serious nutrient depletion. These drugs deplete *calcium* by increasing the excretion of calcium in the urine. Calcium depletion causes a greater need for vitamin D which in turn can cause a *vitamin D* deficiency. *Potassium* and *magnesium* are also excreted in larger amounts and depletion of these two nutrients can cause a wide number of issues including dizziness, muscle weakness, irregular heartbeat, edema, excessive thirst, mental and nervous disorders, insomnia, high blood pressure, and osteoporosis. *Zinc, vitamin c, selenium*, and *vitamin A* are also all depleted which increases free radical damage and weakens the immune system. *Chromium* deficiency also occurs which can result in insulin resistance, elevated blood sugar, and high cholesterol. *Vitamin B12* deficiency will cause extreme weakness and depression. Finally, *folic acid* is depleted by corticosteroids as well.

**Aspirin**: This drug causes the substantial depletion of *vitamin C*, as well as *calcium, folic acid, sodium, potassium, iron,* and *vitamin B5*. Lack of iron will cause anemia, brittle nails, hair loss, and a weakened immune system. B5 deficiency is rare since it is so abundant in the diet, however symptoms are fatigue and listlessness.

**Sulfasalazine:** Here is yet another drug that depletes *folic acid*.

**Indomethacin:** Depletes *folic acid* and *iron*. Iron supplementation is usually not recommended unless a lab test determines that there is a deficiency.

**Non-Steroidal Anti- Inflammatory Drugs, or NSAID's:** Deplete, you guessed it, *folic acid* as well as *iron*.

**Hydroxychloroquine, or Plaquenil:** Long term use will cause a decrease in *calcium* and *vitamin D*, both vital in skeletal health.

**Tetracyclines:** All antibiotics will affect gastrointestinal health by killing off beneficial bacteria in the gut. These bacteria work to manufacture and absorb a number of vitamins. They also prevent the overgrowth of yeast and other harmful organisms in the body. Tetracylines will deplete the full range of *B vitamins* and *vitamin K* which are produced by beneficial bacteria, as well as *magnesium, calcium, zinc*, and *iron*. Whenever taking antibiotics it is important to supplement with probiotics after short term use and during long term use.

**Amitriptyline (Elavil):** This drug is sometimes used to help insomnia in arthritis and can result in decreased *vitamin B2 (riboflavin),* and *coenzyme Q10. Coenzyme Q10* is very important in the health of our cells and isn't abundant in food. It is manufactured in the cells and is important in energy production in the mitochondria. It also protects heart and circulatory health and is a powerful antioxidant. *Riboflavin* is important in the health of the skin, eyes, and mucus membranes as well as metabolism of food, energy, growth, and reproduction.

**Azathooprine (Imuran):** This immune suppressant drug depletes *niacin.*

**Penacillamine (Cuprimine, Depen):** The list of depleted nutrients for this drug includes *copper, zinc, iron, magnesium*, and *vitamin B6*, which is necessary for the function of over sixty enzymes. Deficiency of B6 can result in insomnia, PMS, elevate heart disease risk, depression, nervousness, anemia, nausea, and lethargy. Copper deficiency can result in fatigue, anemia, increased cholesterol, and decreased connective tissue repair.

**Cyclophosphamide (Cytoxan):** Depletion of *vitamin E* occurs with high doses of this drug.

This obviously isn't a comprehensive list, but it hopefully is enough to make you realize that nutrition is vitally important for people who are taking medications. By being diligent and making sure you are feeding your body quality, nutritious foods you will be able to ward off some side effects to medications while you improve your general health and well being.

So, how about a list of foods high in some of the nutrients commonly depleted with arthritis medications?

| Coenzyme Q10 | Folic Acid | Magnesium | Calcium | Vitamin E |
|---|---|---|---|---|
| Mackerel | Barley | Blackstrap Molasses | Salmon | Leafy Vegetables |
| Salmon | Lentils | Seafood | Sardines | Brown Rice |
| Sardines | Bran | Avocados | Leafy Vegetables | Wheat Germ |
| | Chicken | Apples | Broccoli | Oatmeal |
| | Leafy Vegetables | Figs | Yogurt | Pinto Beans |
| | Wheat Germ | Nuts | Parsley | Peas |
| | Salmon | Sesame Seeds | Asparagus | Wheat Germ |
| | Whole Grains | Millet | Sesame Seeds | Spinach |
| | Cauliflower | | | Sweet Potatoes |
| | | | | Cold Pressed Vegetable Oils |
| | | | | Nuts |

| Riboflavin | Iron | Zinc | Potassium | Vitamin K |
|---|---|---|---|---|
| Beans | Oysters | Fish | Fish | Broccoli |
| Eggs | Clams | Legumes | Avocados | Leafy Vegetables |
| Milk | Tofu | Pumpkin Seeds | Figs | Brussel Sprouts |
| Spinach | Almonds | Sunflower Seeds | Sunflower Seeds | Cabbage |
| Avocados | Avocados | Mushrooms | Wheat Bran | Oatmeal |
| Broccoli | Beets | Pecans | Yams | |
| Asparagus | Dates | Whole Grains | Raisins | |
| Currants | Blackstrap Molasses | | | |
| Nuts | Pears | | | |
| | Millet | | | |
| | Soybeans | | | |

## *Special Diets*

You don't have to live with rheumatoid arthritis long these days before someone will tell you about a special diet they have heard about that helps to improve symptoms. As you've been gathering throughout this chapter, diet and arthritis are linked, but as with everything related to this disease, there isn't a finite link between the two that is a common thread for everyone. There are a lucky few who discover that they have a food allergy that creates arthritis. I say lucky because these people have something concrete to deal with that will alleviate their symptoms. And I'm sure that there is a grandpa out there who started drinking gin soaked raisins and was dancing the jig the next day. Hooray for them I say and I truly mean it. However, for the rest of us it's best to keep in mind that these are individual cases, and with all individuals what works for one person may or may not work for the next.

This being said, I'm going to mention some interesting research about the issue of diet and rheumatoid arthritis.

One study reported in the Annals of Rheumatic Diseases compared 73 people who developed a form of rheumatoid arthritis and 143 who didn't and looked at their diet over an eight year period. The people who developed arthritis ate less fruits and vegetables and those that consumed the least amount of vitamin C had three times the risk. Those that consumed the least amount of fruits and vegetables had twice the risk [48]

Another study demonstrated that an anti-inflammatory diet with or without supplementation with fish oil significantly reduced symptoms in people with active arthritis [49]

A two week pilot study compared a group of individuals with active rheumatoid arthritis, either giving them prednisone or putting them on an elemental diet (grain, lactose, and sugar free). The diet was just as effective as 15 mg of prednisone at improving both subjective and objective measures of disease activity. [50]

People with a genetic susceptibility to sensitivity to gluten or lectins, a dietary protein, may develop arthritis as nutrient absorption malfunctions and food sensitivities are triggered with the consumption of foods containing these substances. Lectins are found in wheat, barley, oats, corn, and legumes. Gluten is found in the grains wheat, barley, rye and oats. Specifically, those who followed a vegan, gluten free diet for a year showed significant improvements suggesting that reactivity to food antigens can play a role in sustaining arthritis.[51]

*Arthritis Today* magazine reported in March, 2008 that food sensitivities and arthritis were linked in a study from Oslo, Norway. Researchers examined the intestinal fluid of people with and without arthritis and found higher levels of antibodies to cow's milk, pork, codfish, cereal, and hen's eggs in those with arthritis.

Many naturopathic doctors and other holistic medical practitioners will recommend an elimination diet to their clients. This entails eating a simple whole food diet of fruits, vegetables, and proteins while eliminating common food allergens like wheat, soy, corn, and dairy. After a period of time these foods are reintroduced and symptoms are monitored. If symptoms get worse when a food is reintroduced it can be deduced that the person is allergic to that food. Given the amount of research out there hinting at an allergic connection I would recommend that everyone try this.

The alkaline diet is another intriguing idea, which to me has a lot of merit. All food leaves a residue after being metabolized that is either acidic or alkaline depending upon the composition of the food, as well as how the person digests it. Because the body needs an alkaline environment to function properly, too much acidity can deplete alkaline reserves (calcium, magnesium, sodium, potassium, iron, and manganese) and contribute to disease. Interestingly, these reserves are some of the very minerals that drugs for arthritis deplete which is why drugs are very acidic. If you are feeling severely depleted it is always a good idea to shift your diet toward more alkaline foods. The goal is an

80/20 ratio of alkaline/acidic foods. More information about this can be found in a number of good books on the subject.

Here is a list of the most alkaline and most acidic foods:

| Alkaline | Acidic |
| --- | --- |
| Lemons | Artificial Sweeteners |
| Watermelon | Sugar |
| Cantaloupe | Lamb |
| Cayenne | White Flour |
| Papaya | Drugs |
| Parsley | Carbonated Beverages |
| Asparagus | Beef |
| Limes | Pastries and Cakes |
| Dates | |

The fact is that up to eighty percent of the immune system is in the gut. This makes sense given the potential there for invasion by harmful substances whether they are parasites, viruses, fungi, or bacteria. We all require a significant quantity of food and liquid every day and most of us eat at least three times a day. Compare that with other potential places for invaders to enter (nose, skin, etc.) and you'll once again wonder at the wisdom of our bodies. From a pure survival standpoint, the logical thing to do is to place the most defenses in the places that are the most vulnerable and where there are the largest amounts of potentially harmful substances. Before food was pasteurized, sanitized, homogenized and washed, there were a lot more bad guys hanging out on our food and even now, with the occasional outbreaks of salmonella, staphylococcus, etc. from food we are reminded that we our vulnerable at times to infection from the foods we eat.

For me this answers the question of why connections between food allergies and arthritis are found in study after study. This is also why I feel that along with focusing on what I eat it's just as important to enhance how I digest my food. I know that if my digestion is strong it will do what it's supposed to do, which is to absorb water, breakdown the food I eat, assimilate all of the wonderful nutrients it contains, and prevent the infiltration of toxins into my system. On the other hand if my digestion is weak I increase the number of toxins and undigested food particles in my body, thereby increasing the chance of confusing and taxing my immune system.

Enhancing digestion involves, among other things, avoiding food allergens, maintaining a healthy dose of good bacteria by eating fermented foods regularly, supplementing with digestive enzymes when eating cooked or processed foods, and eating slowly, in a relaxed manner and a happy state of mind.

## *Easy Answers are Hard to Come By*

As the plot thickens I hope I haven't discouraged anyone. When it comes to arthritis, I believe that there may be some easy answers out there, but easy answers are hard to come by. Here are some (relatively) easy answers I came by the hard way:

**1. I am what I eat.** As a person with rheumatoid arthritis I know that just like anyone I am what I eat, but I also know that the stakes are higher for me because I already have a larger need for vitamins, minerals, nutrients, and antioxidant and anti-inflammatory foods. My immune system cells are often working in overdrive, and because they are my body is spending a lot of it's time using these substances up, creating the need for more and more. I'm also taxing my liver, kidneys, and other vital organs each time I take a medication, and since for the majority of my life I've done that every day I don't have as much room for other toxins that stress the organs before I'll suffer ill effects. My opinion is that one huge reason people with rheumatoid arthritis have a higher rate of cancers, heart disease, skin reactions, and loss of muscle mass is because we are in a chronically depleted state. As someone with arthritis that has decided to thrive, I know that when I eat whole foods in their natural state I am feeding my body the ingredients of health. I know that when I eat processed foods I am feeding my body substances that it has to work harder to make use of, satiating myself with something that is basically taking up space without doing much good.

**2. I am what I assimilate.** For all of us, what we assimilate into our bodies is the real issue, not what we eat. As a person with rheumatoid arthritis I know that for much of my life my digestive system has been compromised, and I know that I wasn't assimilating the food I ate the way my body desperately needed me to. From the age of two and a half I took baby aspirin. When I got an ulcer at the age of ten, the doctors told me to drink milk and changed my regime to coated aspirin which dissolved in my intestine instead of my stomach. This meant that for years I associated food with discomfort and pain. I've taken drugs that have severely taxed my liver and depleted all of the good bacteria in my gut. For much of my life the food/arthritis link was dismissed, and I was unaware of all of the ways I could have helped my body get beyond these challenges and enhance the absorption of the food I ate.

Knowing what I know now, I've slowly shifted my diet and enjoyed a change in how my body reacts to food. I now add fermented foods into my diet like tempeh, fermented vegetables and raw sauerkraut, which I know will enhance the good bacteria in my colon. I also eat yogurt and whenever I need to take antibiotics for any reason I make sure that I take a probiotic supplement after the course of antibiotics is finished so that I can avoid a leaky gut. I eat raw foods at most every meal so that I'm giving my body the enzymes it needs to fully digest and assimilate what I've eaten, and I don't have to further deplete the enzyme reserves in my organs. I know that by eating some rabbit food as I'm preparing my meal or as an appetizer I'm also doing another great thing for myself, I'm practicing weight control. If I've eaten some raw vegetables early in my meal I won't eat too much later. I eat when I have time to eat, so that I know I can chew and appreciate my food fully.

**3. I am what I enjoy.** I like ice cream. I like cookies. Does that make me a bad person? No, but it can make me a fool if I flagellate myself every time I eat one of these foods knowing that they will never make any healthy food list. French women don't get fat because they enjoy their food. They spend time eating instead of jamming food into their mouths between meetings. They eat chocolate and croissants with their friends without spending the whole time talking about how much they need to go on a diet. Some people say that how you feel about your food is just as important as what's in it for how your body reacts. Negative emotions will always result in negativity. There is no bad food unless you feel bad about it, so stop. Eating some skittles with red dye # 5 won't cause you to keel over and die. Three cookies don't make a person obese. Health never exists on the extreme end of any bell curve and that goes for diet as well. A severe attitude towards any dietary regime that takes the enjoyment out of eating will do more harm than good.

**4. I am what I am.** It may not be politically correct to say this, but looking good does make you feel good. I know that eating well makes my body look better and when I am proud of the way my body looks I am more comfortable in my skin. Speaking for me and my life experience, being comfortable in my skin has always been, and continues to be, one of my top life goals. I'm not always in control of this, especially on days that I'm experiencing pain and swelling, but because I know that when my diet is balanced and healthy my skin looks good, my energy improves, my stomach doesn't hurt, and I stay slim, and this helps to minimize the impact of those challenging days. People who at their core feel good about themselves will make better food choices and end up healthier; people who don't end up in patterns of emotional eating. Emotional eaters end up overeating, undereating, or making poor food choices to fill an emotional need. People who restrict their food are unconsciously trying to exert control over a situation that overwhelms them. If you find yourself doing this it is important to get help with managing your feelings as soon as possible. If you don't you'll be setting yourself up for a spiral down into a pattern of disordered eating or an eating disorder which can be hard to climb back out of. People who overeat are filling an emotional need as well. Every behavior has a reason, so if you find yourself in a pattern of overeating try to notice what triggers this behavior. Then you'll be able to come up with ideas about what non food related activities can replace your self-defeating pattern. Bad food choices can be as simple as the adage

"Because it is there," and then turn into self-beratement or criticism every time you eat ice cream instead of a piece of fruit. If you find yourself in this position cleanse your house of all the foods you know will tempt you and replace them with food choices that are good and good for you. Allow yourself an ice cream cone or cookie once in awhile but go to the store and buy one serving. If that's not possible give the rest away. This way you won't be denying yourself pleasure but you will be taking care of your body. The bottom line with emotional eating is that there is an underlying emotional need that isn't being met and until this is dealt with, you will continue to feel bad about yourself on the inside and end up treating yourself poorly on the outside.

**5. I am an individual.** Cookbook diets, no matter how good they may be, work for the majority of people, but if you happen to fall in the minority you're out of luck. Whenever you decide to make a change in your diet remember above all else to listen to your body and see how it responds. It's quite possible that some foods that promote inflammation for most of us will have the opposite effect on a few folks out there. Ginger may come with five gold stars as an anti-inflammatory herb, but just like any herb some people will use it and proceed to break out in hives.

When it comes to diet and nutrition, the best thing to do is to experiment, take one step at a time, have fun with the process, and feel good about your choices. Think about this, what is your core desire? What is your true motivation for change? Let this be your new mantra when you are shopping for, preparing, and enjoying your food. Let this guide you toward a healthier lifestyle.

## Anti-inflammatory Herbs, Spices, Vitamins, and Minerals

| Herbs & Supplements | Spices | Vitamins & Minerals |
|---|---|---|
| Ginger | Ginger | Vitamin K |
| Yucca | Cinnamon | Vitamin E |
| Turmeric | Cloves | Selenium |
| Grape Seed Extract | Curry | B Vitamins |
| Pycnogenol | Parsley | Zinc |
| Devil's Claw | Garlic | Vitamin C |
| Cat's Claw | Cilantro | Beta Carotene |
| Green Tea | Chives | Germanium |
| Bromelain | Oregano | |
| Boswellia | Rosemary | |
| Feverfew | Turmeric | |
| Elder Leaves and Berries | Basil | |
| Plantain | Cardamom | |
| Oregano | | |
| Quercetin | | |
| Cayenne | | |
| White Willow | | |
| Witch Hazel | | |
| Licorice | | |
| German Chamomile | | |
| Red Clover | | |
| Fish Oils | | |

## *Chapter Five Worksheets*

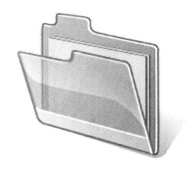

- My Nutrition Worksheet
- One Month Dietary Change Plan

# MY NUTRITION WORKSHEET

1. How will I increase the omega 3 fatty acids in my diet?_____
_____
_____

2. How will I minimize processed foods in my diet? How will I replace them with whole grains?
_____
_____

3. How will I increase the variety of fruits and vegetables I eat? Can I incorporate more organic foods into my diet?_____
_____
_____

4. How will I incorporate helpful spices into my diet?_____
_____
_____

5. Are there any supplements that I want to add to my diet? What are they? _____
_____
_____

6. Do I want to investigate food allergies? What is my plan to do this?_____
_____
_____

7. Which anti-inflammatory foods will I eat more of?_____
_____
_____
_____

Here Are Five Foods That I Will Limit Or Avoid:
1._____
2._____
3._____
4._____
5._____

Here are Five Foods That I will Eat More Of:
1._____
2._____
3._____
4._____
5._____

What is my core desire? _____
_____
_____
_____
_____

# ONE MONTH DIETARY CHANGE PLAN

Week 1: One dietary change I will make this week is: _____
_____
_____
_____

Did I reach this goal? If not, why not?_____
_____
_____
_____
_____


Week 2: One dietary change I will make this week is: _____
_____
_____
_____

Did I reach this goal? If not, why not?_____
_____
_____
_____


Week 3: One dietary change I will make this week is: _____
_____
_____
_____

Did I reach this goal? If not, why not?_____
_____
_____
_____


Week 4: One dietary change I will make this week is: _____
_____
_____
_____

Did I reach this goal? If not, why not?_____
_____
_____
_____

*Someone once told me that I acted like a shark, afraid that if I stopped moving I would die. Most sharks will literally die if they stop swimming: the comparison was more apt than I wanted to admit. At the time I was in remission from the arthritis and living in a small town in Colorado where the mountains were always beckoning me. That summer I had decided I was going to do the Courage Classic, a multi-day bike ride to raise money for Children's Hospital in Denver that would take me over many mountain ranges and many, many miles on the road. The shortest ride I'd do was 50 miles and the longest was just over 100. I found myself training just about every day with some other folks in my town meeting after work to ride up to the base of Wolf Creek Pass.*

*I felt free and happy. On my bike I was strong and for once the arthritis wasn't holding me back. On the days I wasn't riding with my new fast friends I headed up the hills behind my house. I came to know every nook and cranny of those trails until I could ride them backwards blindfolded.*

*Working and biking had become my life and it felt good. I remembered back to when I first had moved out West and dreamed of actually completing a Century Ride, a full 100 miles, thinking that would be the highlight of my life. I had daydreams of being featured in the newspaper and would imagine the headline, "Young woman who beat the odds of arthritis on her bike." When I finally did accomplish that goal there weren't any marching bands or fireworks to greet me and I just hungered for more. The next goal became to do a Century Ride every summer. Then, to do a Century and the Courage Classic.*

*The weekend of the ride we drove up to Leadville, Colorado into cloudy skies and cold, damp weather. I ignored the aches that started to creep into my joints. On the second day, the day that we would ride 104 miles up two mountain passes, my pain had started to settle in. My good friend Tim, a lanky red head who was born for the bike had taken it upon himself to look after me and he told the shuttle car (a van that will pick you up if you get too tired to ride) to stay close. Time and again the van driver would drive up to next us and ask, "Need a ride?" and I'd quickly shout, "NO!" Then Tim, who'd been to the top of the mountain at least once, would ride back down and say to me, "You should take the shuttle, this is a really long ride and you are suffering too much."*

*My response was anger. I railed at Tim and said he had no right to tell me what to do. I told him to stop telling the driver I needed a ride. He didn't listen and it became a battle of wills. My anger spurred me up the hill and to the end in driving rain. Tim and I patched things up later that summer but he never knew why I was really angry. I wasn't angry at him, I was angry at myself for being the "weak" one. My fantasy of the bike as the equalizer had been dismantled and the shadow of the arthritis was chasing me down. I had to prove to myself that I could beat it.*

*So I kept riding. All summer, into the fall, just like the postman I'd ride in rain, snow, sleet, or hail. This made for some exciting stories but I was too busy riding to see that I was the only one so seemingly possessed. Even Tim, who'd been a bike racer, didn't feel the need to put in the hours I did. Why was I doing this? Not because I was like a shark and thought if I stopped I'd die, but because I was afraid if I stopped the arthritis would be there to greet me. When finally it did it wasn't because I had stopped but because I hadn't stopped enough.*

*My history with exercise began as I grew up in a suburban town in the 70's and 80's, before Amber alerts and driving your kids to school became the norm. We walked everywhere, to school, our friend's houses, into town. On weekends we were told to, "Get out of the house and play with your friends, be back for dinner," and we were happy to do so. Spring meant softball season, summer, swimming and camping, Fall was for raking the leaves into huge piles and jumping into them and taking bike trips to Vermont, and finally, Winter was ski season.*

*An idyllic picture except for one thing; my arthritis tended to get in the way of the fun. I was, and still am, someone who loves to be active and has a hard time sitting out of anything so I figured out how to keep up. That meant hiding my pain, never complaining, and learning to numb myself. Except for the last part, this was actually not hard to do because none of the kids that surrounded me had a clue about what I was enduring and the adults didn't seem to notice. In junior high I was on the basketball team with my best friend and managed to keep up in practice but was a bit out of my league during the games. I was quite happy to be the bench warmer until we were twenty points ahead. Being a full head shorter than everyone else put a damper on my dreams of being the next Magic Johnson, but as long as I was part of things I felt happy. My arthritis was a considerable bother but I managed to keep my pain in check by grinning and bearing it so I could hide it from the other kids and keep the adults in the dark. Inside though I watched how the other kids moved with ease, not having to think about kneeling or jumping. They were blissfully unaware that I watched them and compared their ease with my careful planning just about every move I made to keep the pain to a minimum.*

*Then came high school. The one extracurricular activity that I had was sports and in high school there wasn't room for someone like me on the team. All my friends were star players and without them to hang out with I felt part of my identity was gone. So I withdrew. I became a straight A student and then a girl with anorexia. As with everyone who endures anorexia knows, the causes are complicated and unique. For me, the anorexia was in part a solution to my new identity problem. If I couldn't be a good athlete at least I could be thin. I knew my Dad admired thinness because he was always worried about my older sister's weight. I had always been the skinny one and I intended to stay that way despite the onset of puberty and the effects of the estrogen pills that I had to go on after an episode of almost bleeding to death when I first started menstruating. Around this time I stopped exercising because I had no energy, something that will happen when you are starving yourself.*

*Years later I rediscovered how fun it was to move my body and feel strong. When I moved out West, exercise became a part of my life again, this time on my own terms. Gone were basketball, softball, tennis, and swimming in cold water. Instead I started to bike. Which led to the day of the Courage Classic.*

*It took many years and a monster flare up that took me away from that beautiful remission to look at why being active is so important to me. I had to do this because I found that in an active disease state, the ramifications of overdoing it are so much larger than when you don't have inflamed joints.*

*Here's what I've come to realize:*
*It's okay to love being active, it's okay to want to climb mountains and ride 100 miles on my bike. It's also okay to envy people when I see them move their bodies effortlessly in ways that I never will because of my pain and fused joints. It's okay to feel thwarted at times in my attempts to live life to its fullest. It's okay to do something I really want to even though I know I may pay for it later because it brings me joy. It's okay to sit one out.*

*It's not okay to punish myself by pushing so hard that I make myself worse just to prove my worth. It's not okay to identify myself with what I am capable of doing on a particular day. It's not okay to think less of myself because I limp sometimes. It's not okay to blame myself for any of this even if I did screw up here and there. Life is for learning and you learn as you go.*

*These days, whenever I'm out hiking in the woods near my home and my joints are talking to me loudly I make myself*

183

*think of people who aren't able to move at all. My frustration will melt a bit and turn into determination and gratitude. I remember that even though my body creates pain that I feel gets in my way, it also simultaneously works incredibly hard to move me up that hill.*

*For me, thinking about the millions of nerves, hormones, and chemicals that course through my body to keep me upright and moving forward throughout life is mind boggling and humbling at the same time. The arthritis may be something going "wrong" with me but there is also so much that is going right. In my opinion I don't have to go searching to believe in miracles, all I really need to do is look in the mirror. Having arthritis is a constant reminder not to take that miracle for granted and instead to take responsibility and honor it. This means that I need to do whatever I can to help my body, my miracle, function well.*

*I've realized that the key to honoring your body's needs is to actually listen to it. I've spent much of my life tuning it out because I didn't like what I heard or saw and this hurt me in more ways than one. It turned my relationship with myself into a battlefield and I was always the casualty. Lately I've been trying to tune into my body instead of tuning it out when I exercise and it's been interesting what I've been hearing. I've learned that it really likes to move but it also needs a lot more rest than I ever have given it. I've learned that when I honor my body it honors me back, and that lesson is priceless.*

## Chapter Six:
Exercise, Making Moving a Part of Your Life

> *"Movement is a medicine for creating change in a person's physical, emotional, and mental states. "*
>
> *-Carol Welch, movement educator*

Expert opinions regarding exercise and arthritis have swung from one end of the spectrum to the other. Not so long ago a person in a flare up was put in a hospital and then sent home to bed. Exercise was avoided; instead people were strapped into all kinds of splints to hold their joints in place and given range of motion exercises so they wouldn't completely stiffen up. These days exercise is encouraged and research has shown the numerous benefits of exercise for improving bone density, function, mood, and overall quality of life in people with arthritis.

The question is no longer, "Should I exercise?" Instead it's, "What should I do?" Unfortunately, only 15% of people with arthritis exercise three or more times a week and a whopping 70% don't do any regular physical activity at all. Compare this to the population as a whole 30 % of who exercise regularly and 39 % who don't and you'll see a big difference.[52] Although the general population is doing much better than people with arthritis, both of these statistics leave a lot to be desired. The Center for Disease Control and Prevention recommends at least thirty minutes of moderate physical activity five or more times per week because inactivity puts you at risk for many diseases such as heart disease, diabetes, metabolic syndrome as well as an early death. As many of you know all too well, having arthritis doesn't prevent you from getting something else, so if you want to improve your overall health and decrease your risk for disease, following the CDC's guidelines would be a great place to start.

## *Variety is the Spice of Life*

The questions then become, "What type of exercise is the best for arthritis?" "How do I exercise on my bad days?" and, "How do I know I'm not damaging my joints?" All of these are valid questions that really need to be thought through before you start any exercise program and as you monitor your progress.

So, what type of exercise IS best for rheumatoid arthritis? The general answer is non-weight bearing exercises like swimming and bike riding which put less strain on the joints. As a comparison, running is high impact and with each foot strike you are bearing two to four times your body weight.

The more specific answer is that you need to consider which joints are the most affected, as well as any instability in your affected joints, your current level of swelling, and your pain level. Any activity you do that increases your pain for longer than two hours afterwards is not a good one. This is called the *two hour pain rule* and it's been a standard for many years. Since the goal for aerobic exercise is 30-60 minute sessions you need to be relatively comfortable, otherwise you won't last. As for joint instability, it's important to keep in mind where your instabilities are and let pain be your guide. For example, if your fingers are swollen you'll want to avoid rowing machines or racket sports.

Another aspect to this is variety. It is best to have a few different kinds of exercise in your repertoire. Not only will that prevent you from overstraining one joint or group of joints, it will keep you from getting bored. You also want to consider convenience and cost. You don't want any barriers to doing exercise. The most important component of the type of exercise you choose though is that it has to be fun. If it isn't rewarding in some way you aren't going to keep doing it and unless it becomes a part of your life the benefits you gain won't be lasting.

The best way to approach exercise when you have arthritis is realistically. Start where you are and try not to compare yourself in the present with what you were able to do in the past. Progress slowly with small, manageable goals and aim to make exercise a part of your life. Pacing is key; it's important not to push too hard on bad days even if it means you aren't reaching your goal and you definitely don't want to make up for lost days by doubling your activity level when you feel better. Stick with your plan, remember that life is a marathon not a race, and even if you have a bad month there will always be time to reach your goals. Pay attention to the process, not the outcome, and use the opportunity when you are exercising to tune into your body. Along with the pain you may be feeling, try to focus on the parts of your body that are strong. Avoid all or nothing thinking, because it's always better to do a little bit than nothing at all. Make exercise a part of your life by adding activity into your day. It's okay to do three ten minute sessions instead of one thirty minute. Walk more, stretch more, do a bit at a time and gradually you will notice big changes in your body.

## SMART Goals

Exercise goals are very important because they keep you motivated to continue moving forward. Even with the ups and downs of arthritis you can create and reach goals if you follow the acronym SMART: specific, measurable, achievable, relevant, and time-bound.

If a goal isn't **specific** you won't know when you've achieved it. After you write your goal you should be able to answer the question, "How will I know I reached it?" You should be able to **measure** the goal. It can be an internal or an external measure, such as minutes per day, times per week, or a scale of 1 to 10 for internal goals. **Achievable** means realistic. Going back to what I said earlier, start where you are and try not to compare your past with your present. **Relevant** means that it's important to you. You want to create an active life that makes you happy and fits into the picture of who you want to be, not what anyone else expects of you. **Time-bound** means that you set a date to accomplish your goal. This will give you a sense of completion, a huge boost to your self esteem and help you to see the results of your determination and effort.

## Balanced Exercise

Aerobic exercise is only one component of an overall program that also includes resistance training, flexibility, and balance. All of these are important to improving your quality of life, decreasing pain, and preventing more problems from developing.

 Let's look at each one:
*Aerobic exercise* is any exercise that elevates your heart and breathing rate for a sustained period of time. A person who does this form of exercise on a regular basis will be helping their body in a myriad of ways. Resting heart rate goes down, there is an increase in blood flow in the

muscles that are working, calories are expended which decreases body fat, insulin is used more efficiently in the body, overall endurance improves, and the increase in circulation allows nutrition to reach the joints. To get these benefits you need to be exerting yourself at a moderate intensity level. There are two ways to measure this. One is by calculating a heart rate range and then checking your heart rate as you exercise and the other way is by rating your perceived exertion on a scale of 6 to 20. Both are just as effective.

To calculate your heart rate range you first measure your resting heart rate by taking your pulse. Place your index finger on the thumb side of your wrist, palm up. When you feel your pulse count it for 15 seconds and then multiply by 4. This is your resting heart rate. Now, use this equation, called the Karvonen method:

$$(( 220\text{-age}) - RHR) \times \% ) + RHR = EHR$$

**220 - age** is your maximal recommended heart rate
**RHR** is your resting heart rate
**EHR** is your exercise heart rate
**%** is .50 and .85

> *For example, I'm 39, my max heart rate is 181, and my resting heart rate is 65.*
> *((181-65) x .50) + 65 = 123*
> *((181-65) x .85) + 65 = 164*
> *So my heart rate range is 123-164*

For those of you that hate math or don't care to be that precise there is a much easier technique that has been proven to be just as effective. It's called the Borg rate of perceived exertion scale. You rate how hard you are working according to the intensity of your effort, amount of distress, fatigue level, and environment (hot, cold, humid, etc.) This is also great for people with rheumatoid arthritis because these factors have a lot to do with our ability to exercise.

Here's what it looks like:

| | |
|---|---|
| **6** | **No exertion at all** |
| **7** | **Extremely light** |
| **8** | |
| **9** | **Very light** |
| **10** | |
| **11** | **Light** |
| **12** | |
| **13** | **Somewhat hard** |
| **14** | |
| **15** | **Hard (Heavy)** |
| **16** | |
| **17** | **Very Hard** |
| **18** | |
| **19** | **Extremely Hard** |
| **20** | **Maximal Exertion** |

In general you want to stay between 12 and 15. This will give you a good, moderate workout and help you to stay in your heart rate range.

*Resistance training* is very important for everyone, but in my opinion even more important for people with arthritis. In some ways this appears counterintuitive because it may seem like you are stressing already stressed joints. That may have a ring of truth to it, but then again everyday life stresses joints as well. If you are using joints that aren't supported by strong muscles the risks are even greater.

There are a lot of reasons to do what you can to keep muscles strong. Resistance training will not only help to tone and build muscle, but will also increase your resting metabolism which means that you will burn more calories throughout the day. This is because muscle tissue takes more energy to maintain. The more muscle you have the more calories you will need to consume each day. When you have arthritis, muscle mass declines because during flare ups you aren't able to use your muscles as much without severe pain. As the saying goes, if you don't use it you lose it. The fact is that for every week of bed rest muscle mass decreases ten to fifteen percent. Another reason to consider strength training is the benefit to your bones. Resistance training will increase bone density in the areas that are being worked. Add this to the fact that after age forty-five people generally lose one percent of their muscle mass per year, something called sarcopenia.

Resistance training doesn't have to involve lifting heavy weights. In fact, when you start a program you really want to err on the side of caution if your joints are at all swollen, painful, or unstable. Even one or two pound weights can make a difference to start or you can choose to do exercises that don't involve any equipment at all, called body weight exercises. Ankle or arm weights that can be strapped to your arms may be more joint friendly if your hands are involved. Ideally you want to do eight to ten exercises that move all your major muscle groups including the shoulders, chest, arms, back, abdominals, gluteal muscles, hips, and legs. A personal trainer or physical therapist can guide you when you are starting out to create a customized program to fit your needs; however I'm going to describe basic program to act as a guide.

## Shoulders

The shoulder is an intricate ball and socket joint that has a lot of mobility at the expense of stability. People with rheumatoid arthritis are at higher risk for tears of the small muscles of the shoulder that help to keep the shoulder joint in place, called the rotator cuff muscles.

Here are some exercises that help to strengthen the rotator cuff. These exercises should be done with light weights (no more than four pounds), or no weights at all and you can do each one ten to twenty times, up to three sets

- *Shoulder extension*: Lie on a flat surface, face down and one arm hanging down off the side. With palm facing forward and arm straight, lift the arm back and up towards your body, breathing out. When your arm is parallel to your body hold for three seconds, then breathe in and relax down.

- *Shoulder abduction*: Returning to your original position, arm hanging down and palm facing forward, lift your arm out to the side. Breathe out and keep your arm straight. Hold for three seconds and then breathe in and relax your arm down.

- *Shoulder external/internal rotation*: Sitting upright, bend your elbows ninety degrees so they are parallel to the floor with your hands in front of you. Keep elbows in to your sides and move your hands back as far as is comfortable. You will feel your shoulder blades come together. Breathe out and hold this position for three seconds. Breathe in and come back to center.

- *Shoulder Flexion*: Seated or standing, arms hanging down by your side and palms facing back, breathe out and bring your arms straight up in front of you until they reach shoulder height. Hold, then breathe in and relax down.

## Elbows/Forearms

- *Elbow extension*: Lie on a flat surface and with hands shoulder width apart and facing each other, straighten your arms. Now, breathe in and bend the elbows, then breathe out and straighten.

- *Elbow flexion*: Sitting or standing and arms at your side, palms in, breathe out and bend the elbows, breathe in and straighten. This can be done with palms facing down or up.

- *Forearm internal/external rotation*: Still seated, let your hands relax down by your side. Now, rotate your hand so the palm faces forward then back.

## Hands

There are twenty-seven bones and almost as many joints in each hand, many of which are prone to arthritis. The flexor muscles in the fingers, the muscles that help you make a fist, are naturally ten times stronger that the extensor muscles, or those that straighten your fingers. When hands hurt the tendency is to hold them with the fingers bent so it is very important to try to keep all you hand muscles as balanced as possible by working the smaller, weaker muscles. These exercises don't involve weights and can be done anytime, so they are good to do whenever you think of it throughout the day.

- *Finger "Tap dancing"*: Tap your fingers on a table or your lap one at a time and try to lift them as high as you can as you do this.

- *Finger "Walking"*: Place palms flat on a hard surface, and then slide each finger, one by one, towards the thumb.

- *Finger "Table"*: Hold hands in front of you, palms facing each other and fingers straight. Keeping fingers straight bend at the knuckles, then straighten. Next, keep knuckles straight and bend the top two joints, and then straighten.

- *Wrist circles*: With hands in front of you make wrist circles, keeping your movement slow and the circles as wide as you can manage.

## Chest

Chest exercises are called multi-joint because they involve two or more joints being moved at once.

- *Chest Press*: Lie on your back and place your arms above the chest with palms facing out. Breathe in and bend elbows, lower arms until your upper arms are parallel to the floor and your forearms are parallel to each other. Breathe out and straighten arms, don't lock the elbows.

## Back

Keeping the back strong is very important, especially for people who are prone to low back pain.

- *Back extension*: Lie on your stomach and place your hands under your forehead. Breathe out and lift your upper body off the floor, squeezing the lower back muscles. Make sure you are moving the upper body as a unit and that you feel the low back muscles working. Breathe in and lower.

## Abdominals

The benefit of strengthening the stomach muscles is more than aesthetic, it will help you to breathe deeper and give you a strong core which will make all movement easier.

- *Crunches*: Lie on your back with your feet on the floor. Place hands on your chest, contract your stomach muscles, and bring your head, neck, and shoulders up off the floor, breathing out. Don't strain your neck; remember to work from your core. Breathe in and relax down.

- *Reverse crunches*: Lie on your back with your knees bent and lower legs parallel to the floor. Breathe in and bring feet down to the floor, then breathe out and raise them back up. Don't let your back arch as you do this.

## Hips/ Thighs

The hips, like the shoulders, are ball and socket joints that have a lot of flexibility and are very important in maintaining overall lower body function.

- *Wall sit*: Stand, leaning against a wall. Let your body slide down, until your thighs are parallel to the floor and then hold this position for twenty to sixty seconds. Remember to breathe the entire time.

- *Leg raise*: Stand where you can hold onto a counter or table top. Lift one leg out to the side with your foot flexed and your leg straight, breathing out. Hold this position for three seconds then relax down and breathe in. Switch sides.

- *Kick back*: Still standing, face the counter and bring one leg straight back. Hold, and then relax down.

- *Thigh squeeze*: Lie on your back and hold an exercise ball between your lower legs. You can also use any kind of lightweight ball if you don't have an exercise ball. Squeeze your inner thighs together and hold for three seconds, then relax.

- *Hip Lift*: Lie on your back with feet flat on the floor. Lift your back off the floor slowly, one vertebrae at a time, until you are in a bridge position with your body in a straight line from your knees to your neck. Hold for three seconds, and then relax down.

## Lower Legs
- *Step Up*: Standing on a step or platform step down to the ground, then up.
- *Heel raises*: Stand on a step or platform and bring feet back until your heels are free. Holding onto a chair or rail for support, breathe out and rise up onto your toes, then back down as far as you can feeling the stretch in your calf. Breath in, hold for three seconds and repeat.

## Ankles and Toes
Keeping ankles and toes as strong and mobile as possible, despite any changes that arthritis has created to the their structure, will do a lot to diminish pain in the area that bears the weight of our entire body.

- *Towel curls*: Sitting with your feet on the floor, with a towel underneath them, lift your toes then curl them and grasp the towel, bunching it up as you continue to lift and curl.

- *Side to side*: Still seated with the towel under one foot, slowly slide the towel back and forth with your foot. Repeat on the other side.

- *Ball roll*: Seated, take a ball and place it under one foot. Slowly roll it back and forth, and then repeat on the other side.

- *Toe squeeze*: Place soft foam toe spacers between your toes. Squeeze your toes together, then release.

All of these exercises will help to start an overall body strengthening program and are arthritis friendly as long as you respect your pain and don't try to lift too much weight before you are ready. There are different strategies for weight lifting depending on your goals (Strengthening, muscle endurance, or building muscle). Strengthening and muscle building involve lifting heavier weights with less repetitions and endurance involves lifting lighter weights with more repetitions. People with arthritis should always start with an endurance program and only move on if their joints have no inflammation or pain when performing exercises.

With all exercise you want to maintain, and if possible, improve your range of motion so a stretching and flexibility program is important to do along with a resistance program. The last thing you need is to build muscle at the expense of movement. Let's talk more about this.

As I said earlier, pain means you are moving less. Not only will this weaken your muscles but it will decrease flexibility. When a person is in pain they will automatically will hold the painful area in a position of comfort which immobilizes the area. Unfortunately, it only takes eight hours of this for muscle fibers to begin to shorten which limits range of motion at the joint. This is why therapists may make night splints to preserve wrist function for people whose wrists are painful.

In order to maintain your flexibility it is important to stretch at least four days a week and daily if possible. Starting at your neck and working down slowly, move each joint as far as it will allow.

Here's a quick list:
- *Neck*: back and forth , circles, side to side

- *Shoulder*: circles, forward and back, back and forward

- *Arms*: up overhead and down, circles

- *Elbows*: up and down , palm up and down

- *Hands and fingers*: up and down, circles, side to side

- *Hips*: circles, side to side, up and down

- *Knees*:  bend and straighten

- *Ankles*: side to side, circles, up and down

I highly recommend joining an exercise group that incorporates flexibility, balance, and strength. There are so many choices these days through the Arthritis Foundation or local community centers so it won't be hard to find one, only hard to choose. My favorite group exercise is Tai Chi, an exercise form from China that is thousands of years old. Tai Chi is practiced all over China by people as young as three and as old as one hundred and three. Regular practice helps balance, strength, and flexibility along with being a lot of fun. There are many Tai Chi forms and even one specifically for arthritis.

Another type of exercise that is becoming popular these days is Pilates. Pilates focuses on strengthening the core, or trunk muscles, the theory being that a strong core improves the entire body's alignment and movement patterns. What isn't as widely known about Pilates is that it was originally developed for bed ridden veterans during World War II and can be adapted for any number of orthopedic conditions. I like this because as someone with two fused wrists, I can't bear weight on my hands which can make some types of exercise, like yoga, a bit frustrating at times.

Pilates, Yoga, Alexander Method, Feldencrais, Tai Chi, and Chi Gung are all forms of mind/body exercise. Each form has a different emphasis but they all encourage you to tune your mind into your body through the use of breathing, awareness, and slow movement. My experience has been that discomfort creates the tendency to disassociate from your body so anything that counteracts that tendency will be of great benefit. I suggest doing some homework about what is available in your area, trying out a few classes, and seeing how you respond to them. It may take awhile to find a class or exercise form that works for you. Sometimes it's a matter of finding the right teacher or recruiting a friend to go with you for motivation.  Be persistent, patient, and have fun with this!

## *Never Say Never*

There will be bad days physically and there will be bad days emotionally. Either way, it's okay to acknowledge to yourself that you wish your life was different. It's okay to throw things and shout your swear words of choice. And then, it's best to do what you can to make yourself feel better. Moving your body any way you can will make you feel better. Incorporating moving into your life will make you function better. It's up to you to make this a priority and fit it into your life.

For most people there will be a type of exercise that is easy to be motivated to do. In my case this is aerobic exercise. There will also be the type that you will find all kinds of excuses not to do. For me this is weight training. Whatever the combination is for you, try to find ways to motivate yourself. This may be joining an exercise group, buying a pedometer and having a goal of walking 5,000 steps a day, or buying yourself something when you've met an exercise goal. Find out what motivates you and use this to reach your goals. Motivate yourself to do something every day and you will find that moving has become part of your lifestyle. You will find that moving is easier. You will find that you are more comfortable in your body. Now THAT is the ultimate goal.

# *Chapter Six Worksheets*

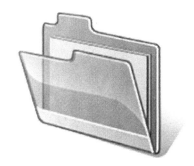

- My Goals
- Exercise Worksheet

# MY GOALS

Specific: _____

_____

_____

_____

_____

_____

_____

_____

_____

_____

_____

_____

How will I know I reached it? _____

_____

_____

## Measurable:

How many times per week, or rated on a scale of 1 to 10?  _____

## Achievable:

Is this goal realistic? Does it leave room for good and bad days?_____

_____

## Relevant:

Why is this goal important to me?_____

_____

_____

_____

_____

## Time Bound:

When will I reach it?_____

_____

_____

_____

_____

_____

# Write your exercise goals here:

_____
_____
_____
_____
_____
_____
_____
_____
_____
_____
_____
_____
_____
_____
_____
_____
_____
_____
_____
_____
_____
_____
_____
_____
_____
_____
_____
_____
_____
_____
_____
_____
_____
_____
_____
_____
_____

# EXERCISE WORKSHEET

How active am I right now?_____

_____

_____

_____

_____

**List all activity that is a part of your life right now.**

House/Yard Work: _____

_____

_____

_____

Job Related: _____

_____

_____

_____

Hobbies:_____

_____

_____

_____

Exercise Routine: _____

_____

_____

_____

List any type of exercise you want to add to your routine: _____

_____

_____

_____

List ways to motivate yourself to do this: _____

_____

_____

_____

What will this add to your life, how will this enhance your life? _____

_____

_____

_____

*I really had no excuse after I graduated from occupational therapy school in my early twenties. I sat through hours of classes discussing joint pathologies, learned about joint protection techniques and body mechanics. I'd even had the opportunity to peer into a real human joint during anatomy class. I knew what I should do. However, I achieved a remission soon after that and was busy proving to myself and the world that arthritis was no longer part of my vocabulary. During this time my life consisted of going full blast until pain or weariness got the best of me and then resting until I could go back at it, all the while berating myself and my body for not performing the way I wanted it to. Looking back, it's a miracle I didn't have a monster flare up before I did. Once the flare up hit I had all the time in the world to stop and make the necessary changes in my habits to move toward remission again.*

*It's not something I woke up one day doing all at once, it's been a process. Changing habits is never easy, especially when you have an emotional attachment to sucking it up and having free will. So I chose to learn the hard way with some things. And I chose to look at why I have an emotional need to keep up. This will be a case of "do as I say, not as I've done," because my process of keeping my joints strong and stable was disorganized at best, but here is what I would have done originally if I could go back and do it all over.*

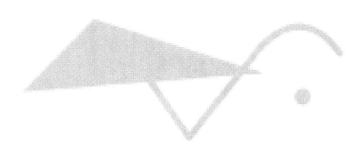

## Chapter Seven:
Keeping Joints Strong and Stable

> *"You have brains in your heads.*
> *You have feet in your shoes.*
> *You can steer yourself any direction you choose."*
> *-Dr. Seuss*

Joint protection is a phrase we've hopefully all heard. Personally, I don't like it because it implies that my joints are fragile and need protected. Regardless of whether they are or not, I prefer not think of them that way. Keeping joints strong and stable is what I am aiming to do and I'm guessing you're with me. I'm also guessing that you've already worked out a number of ways to do this. I never thought about the fact that I push doors open with my forearms and close them with my hip or feet, I just do it. However, there were a number of things I'd always done the hard way until I completely understood why it's so important to keep my joints well positioned as often as possible.

Anytime you put sustained pressure on an inflamed joint you are stretching and pulling on already overstretched tendons and ligaments. You are causing what is called the arthrokinematics, basically the efficient pulley system that causes our joints to move, to misalign. Ultimately, this can result in the dramatic changes to joints that we may have seen or experienced.

If, like me, you've actually experienced joint changes you'll know that at first, when there is prolonged stretching of tissues they become less elastic, more painful, lax, and feel a bit unstable when you use the joint. Eventually, the tissues reshape themselves, certain tendons shrink, others may rupture or just stay stretched and the result is a fixed position that is basically pain free even if it isn't very attractive. The long-term issue with this, besides the cosmetic one, is that changes at one joint will ultimately affect the joints surrounding it, usually putting more strain on them. By the way, this is important to know if you are considering a joint fusion.

## *Avoiding Strain and Pain*

So how do you keep your joints strong and stable? First, become more aware of how you do things. This means getting in touch with your body which is something that is good for everyone. When you do, you'll notice what positions or actions hurt more than others as well as what your body is automatically doing to compensate for the pain.

Compensation usually comes in the form of doing things differently and can be good as long as you keep certain things in mind.

 The goal of compensation is avoidance of strain and pain. Strain and pain usually are the result of using your joints in ways that they can't handle. Let's look at the body and see where healthy compensatory techniques can be useful.  First, at the fingers, you want to limit activities that cause what's called *ulnar deviation*.  Look at your hand. Move the fingers towards the pinky. This is ulnar deviation.  The reason you want to limit this movement is that with long term inflammation in the fingers the tendons that bring the fingers up tend to fall towards the pinky side and then they can become fixed there.

To complicate things, most activities that involve your hand encourage this position.  Pick up a cup, write your name, open the door, carry a bag and you'll see what I mean. Appropriate compensation for this tendency is to use two hands to pick up a cup, or better yet, use light weight drink ware. Use pens that have a large circumference so you're not gripping as tightly, or build them up yourself with cylindrical foam. Install lever style door handles in your house since you'll most likely be using those the most.  Carry bags with your forearms and keep them close to your body. Don't pack bags heavier than you need to, it's better to take two trips into the house.  Here's another tip, open jars with your right hand and close them with your left.  Become aware of things that you do on a daily basis that involve ulnar deviation and learn ways to decrease this tendency. Along with the avoidance of ulnar deviation, using lightweight tools with wide circumferences helps to decrease tight gripping as sustained pressure can quickly result in problems with joint structure and function.

This leads me to the idea that you always want to use bigger joints to complete tasks whenever you can. By placing the forearms close to the body when carrying a load you will avoid stressing the joints.  You can avoid opening doors with your hands by leaning into them with your forearms and your body weight, holding doors open with your foot, or pushing them open with your hips, thighs, or shoulders.  Find and use bags that you can strap across shoulders or use a backpack whenever you need to carry a load for any length of time. Luggage with wheels will save the day when traveling. Instead of a purse, using a fanny pack is also a good idea. Try to avoid heavy lifting whenever possible. If you don't actually have to pick something up and you can wait until someone else is there to help you it's always a good idea. All of these actions will help to keep your body in a more functional position and discourage positions that put increased strain on your joints.

## *Handy Aids*

In addition to the compensatory techniques I just talked about there are numerous gadgets you can get to make life easier. In order to gauge what would be useful to you it's necessary to pay attention to activities you do a lot and those you have difficulty with. Then when you browse through catalogs you'll know what to keep your eyes peeled for.

Here are some of my must haves, as well as some things I do to make my life easier.

### In the kitchen:

- A really good knife

- A U-shaped peeler

- Lightweight cups and mugs

- An automatic can opener

- A jar opener (rubber gloves also work)

- Spring loaded scissors for cutting open cereal pouches, plastic bags etc.

- Keeping a skillet on the stove that I use most often, thus eliminating some heavy lifting

- Storing things that I use most often within easy reach

- Shopping and then preparing my fresh fruit and vegetables by washing and cutting them up. That way, I'll be able to cook a healthy simple meal later and know that I won't have to use a lot of energy to do it.

- Keeping healthy frozen foods available for days that I really have no energy to cook

- Whenever possible I slide, rather than lift, heavy pots and pans across the counter. I also store heavier things so that I can slide them across the counter instead of lifting them.

- I transfer heavy things such as dog food or large containers of milk from big containers to little ones.

**In the living room:**

- Chairs that offer good support are and easy to get in and out of. When purchasing a chair, sit in it and make sure you don't sink down down too far. Look at your knees. Are they higher than your hips? If so, this chair is not for you; it's too much work to get in and out of and over time this adds up.

- A telephone headset to avoid strain on my neck, shoulders, hands, and elbows

**In the bedroom:**

- A really good mattress. In the past, an egg crate mattress cover decreased pain in my shoulders and hips when I slept. I no longer need this because I now have a really good mattress.

- A cervical pillow to keep my neck and shoulders in good alignment as I sleep.

- Scented candles and essential oils that are relaxing to me ( we'll talk more about this in the Sleep chapter)

**In the bathroom:**

- A toothbrush with a wider circumference at the handle

- Smaller containers of a shampoo and conditioner to decrease the strain on my hands

- I also never bother to squeeze out a shampoo and conditioner from their bottle; I just take off the cap and pour. This can take people who shower after me by surprise!

As I said earlier, all of these things didn't happen overnight. It was a very long process for me and had a lot to do with my acceptance that a joint friendly lifestyle was something that needed to be a part of my life.

## *Positioned for Pain*

Along with compensation, when someone is in pain they tend to guard their painful joints. Guarding tenses the muscles around the joint when you're using it so it doesn't hurt so much. The problem with guarding isn't so much that you do it when necessary, it may be the only way you can take that walk and make it through. It's that, more often than not, you will continue to tense those muscles after you've finished with the activity which decreases circulation and nourishment to the tissues. This can result in further degradation of the joint. It may also put the joint in an awkward position for prolonged periods of time, stretching and contracting tissues which is something you definitely want to avoid. One habit that can help with this is tuning into how you are holding your body throughout the day, especially when you're in one position or doing anything for a prolonged time. Take a deep breath, feel where you are holding tension, let it out, and relax. After this, whenever you feel tension do a few gentle range of motion exercises by moving the joint back and forth ten times in a pain-free range. This will further release your tension.

Along with guarding, people with inflamed joints tend to hold their bodies in what's called a position of comfort. This position is often not a functional one and can often end up being detrimental in the long-term to your general health by creating more asymmetry and stressing healthy joints to the point that they may end up with issues as well. We all do this in varying degrees, arthritis or not. The neck and upper back pain many people get when they are stressed is from prolonged hunching of the shoulders.

Think of this multiplied by 2, 4, 6, whatever the number of involved joints you have and you can end up with a lot of pain and stressed tissues. Then consider the danger of performing all of the movements people inevitably do numerous times throughout the day like lifting, pushing, pulling, reaching, or standing when you are guarding, resting in positions of comfort, and have muscle weakness from prolonged arthritis. When you do this you are adding insult to injury and setting yourself up for the possibility of a further trauma. So, let's weed through this mire to come up with how to minimize risks to your already stressed body.

## *Positioned For Health*

Once again, awareness of how your body is reacting to the pain is the first key to what is called body mechanics. It may help at first to purchase a watch with a timer and every thirty minutes or so have it go off to remind yourself to do this.  It will surprise you how quickly you can learn to listen. This will also help you to understand what your positions of comfort are.  Do you keep your elbows held into your body?  Do you tend to keep your ankles turned in?  How are you holding your wrists?

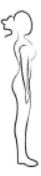

Understanding what a well-balanced body position looks like is a good place to start.

*Notice that weight is evenly distributed and the body is held over the mid feet.  The spine is positioned in a slight S curve.*

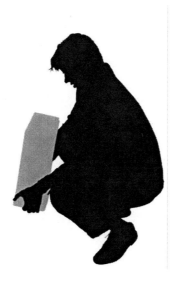

**Correct lifting**

*Knees bent, object held close to body, breathing, back straight and not twisting, using abdominal muscles.*

Whether it's lifting, pushing, or pulling,  remember to use big joints, keep your back aligned, breathe through the activity, bend your knees slightly, pivot your feet instead of twisting at  the back, and stay close to the object. When you practice doing things this way you will have the added benefit of strengthening muscles in a more balanced way.

 Which brings me to my last suggestion, keeping your body as fit as possible.  By maintaining and improving strength in your body you will definitely be placing less stress on your joints. This will also help you to keep your weight down which, if this is an issue for you, further compounds the stress on your joints. If you need incentive to lose weight try walking around with ten pounds strapped to your ankles or wrists and you'll realize how much extra stress you feel on your joints.

Other aspects to keeping joints strong and stable are conserving your energy as much as possible and simplifying daily tasks wherever you can. The best way to begin doing this is by taking stock of your roles and responsibilities. What is required of you on a daily basis?  What activities are physically difficult for you to perform?  What activities are very tiring for you to perform?  Are there activities that may be easy physically, but emotionally draining to you or stressful?

 It's also important to keep in mind that you have a certain amount of energy each day and you need to use it wisely. This means that you're not using all your energy doing things that you have to do and leaving no energy for things that you enjoy or find fun. To reiterate a concept that I learned from one of my favorite self-help gurus, Caroline Myss, try to imagine that every day each person is given 100 energy units and they have to decide how they want to spend it.  When you have rheumatoid arthritis you will be spending quite a bit of internal energy dealing with pain which will be using up a lot of those units. Pain uses up a lot more energy than you think and you really need to be smart about how you use your precious energy.

This is where learning to plan ahead becomes useful.  I love to be a spontaneous person but it's just not practical or really worth it the majority of the time. When you are planning your day or week remember to pace yourself, alternate difficult and easy tasks and activities that require different body positions. Start to slowly make changes to your daily routine, purchase the items that may help make things easier, and learn to delegate. I never open a new jar if there's someone with strong hands around me! You'll be amazed at what small changes can do to make your life so much better. Last but not least, learn to build in speed bumps throughout the day, which means taking time for rest breaks. Napping is a great way to do this. This is especially true when you have more difficult tasks to do that day.

Let's wrap up by giving you an easy way of keeping all this information straight. Think about what putting stress on the joints can do - DISABLE. Take away the DIS and you have ABLE.

## A- Awareness
## B- Body Mechanics
## L-Learn to Pace Yourself
## E- Energy Conservation

# *Chapter Seven Worksheets*

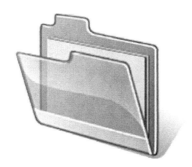

- Balance Wheel
- Balancing My Life
- Learn to be A.B.L.E.

# BALANCE WHEEL

Look at this wheel and think about how happy you are in each of these six areas of your life. Rank each area between 1 to 10, 1 being completely unsatisfied and 10 being completely satisfied.  Now with a marker, fill in each area.  **How balanced is your life?**

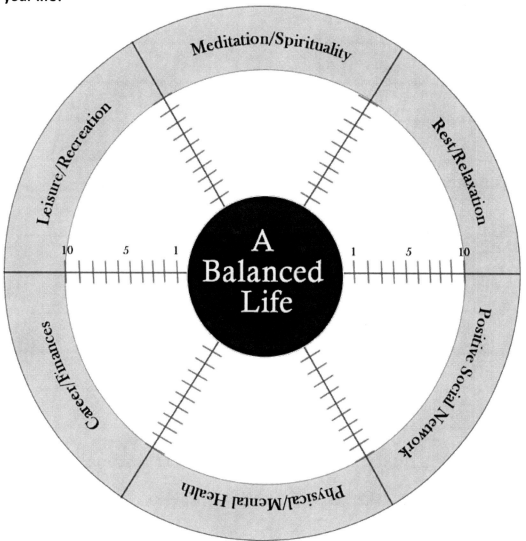

# BALANCING MY LIFE

List all your daily activities, rate them on a scale of 1-10 according to level of enjoyment, and label the ones that are physically demanding or mentally stressful (PD, MS)

| Activity | Enjoyment 1-10 | (PD), (MS) |
|---|---|---|
| 1. | | |
| 2. | | |
| 3. | | |
| 4. | | |
| 5. | | |
| 6. | | |
| 7. | | |
| 8. | | |
| 9. | | |
| 10. | | |
| 11. | | |
| 12. | | |
| 13. | | |
| 14. | | |
| 15. | | |
| 16. | | |
| 17. | | |

**( -)  1**                    **And then place them on this scale**                    **(+) 10**
_____neutral_____

Next, use a different highlighter and highlight the items on the left according to things you have to do, and things you could delegate if you need to. The idea is to tip the scale as much to the right as possible. Finally, Plan. Where will your speed bumps go? Which activities can you use compensatory techniques for to make them easier? Where will better body mechanics make a difference? This close examination will lead you to a healthier, more balanced life.

*How balanced can you be?*

Job to delegate:_____ Who will I delegate to?_____
How will I do this?_____
_____
_____

Job to delegate:_____ Who will I delegate to?_____
How will I do this?_____
_____
_____

Job to delegate:_____ Who will I delegate to?_____
How will I do this?_____
_____
_____

Job to delegate:_____ Who will I delegate to?_____
How will I do this?_____
_____
_____

Job to delegate:_____ Who will I delegate to?_____
How will I do this?_____
_____
_____

Job to delegate:_____ Who will I delegate to?_____
How will I do this?_____
_____
_____

Job to delegate:_____ Who will I delegate to?_____
How will I do this?_____
_____
_____

Job to delegate:_____ Who will I delegate to?_____
How will I do this?_____
_____
_____

Job to delegate:_____ Who will I delegate to?_____
How will I do this?_____
_____
_____

Job to delegate:_____ Who will I delegate to?_____
How will I do this?_____
_____
_____

# LEARN TO BE A.B.L.E.

How will I be more **Aware** of how I do things to compensate for my pain? _____

_____

_____

_____

_____

_____

_____

How will I incorporate correct **Body Mechanics** into my daily activities?_____

_____

_____

_____

_____

_____

_____

How can I **Learn to Pace** myself during the day? What is my plan for this? _____

_____

_____

_____

_____

_____

_____

How will I conserve my **Energy** during the day? Where will my speed bumps go? _____

_____

_____

_____

_____

_____

_____

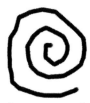

*I grew up in a conservative, middle class suburban town, when what we now call alternative or complementary medicine was associated with "California hippies." The closest I ever came to trying out an unconventional remedy for my arthritis was my daily Flintstone vitamin which tasted so good I decided to take the whole bottle one day. Perhaps a foreshadowing of my future headlong foray into alternative therapy.*

*Because of my upbringing I wasn't exposed to anything but conventional medicine until the age of twenty-five when I moved to Salt Lake City and started to shop at the local Wild Oats, a health food store. There I encountered an amazing array of joint formulas, inflammation eradicators, detoxification mixes, green juices, as well as a lot of well meaning people who took it upon themselves to give me advice about how to take care of my arthritis. This was a whole new world for me and my curious mind was a sponge lapping up all the information I was learning. I tried some of the more intriguing supplements that were recommended to me and had mixed results. One herb relieved a two year case of swollen glands and sore throat but another, touted as a "blood detoxer," made me sick as a dog. I guess I wasn't ready for that after so many years of aspirin and hot dogs. I happily kept dabbling with my new found hobby while I dutifully followed the doctor's orders. Until, gradually my body stopped tolerating my drug regime and I began to suffer with side effect after side effect.*

*Finally my Mom convinced me to go to the Mayo Clinic, the shining star of modern medicine. The plane to Rochester was filled with potential patients including an Arab sheik, and I thought to myself, "Maybe this will be it, I'll finally get some answers." When I got there I saw a rheumatologist who farmed me out to a dermatologist to investigate my severe itchy reactions, a gynecologist to discover why I wasn't menstruating, and a gastroenterologist to find the source of my stomach aches. The dermatologist gave me steroid cream, the gynecologist suggested birth control pills, and the gastroenterologist tested for colitis and found that nothing was wrong. Here I was consulting the best medical minds in the country and this is all they could come up with? I had taken the time, gone the extra mile to find the best medical care this country has to offer and I was left with just as much discomfort and suffering as I had before. I didn't know whether to be angry, distraught, confused, hopeless, or all four.*

*This is when, after so many years of trusting my doctors and following their orders, my disillusionment with medical doctors started. I began a see-saw ride, jumping from conventional medicine to alternative medicine and back searching for a cure. I realized that doctors were ill-equipped to deal with some of my more elusive symptoms, especially when they didn't fit the formal description of rheumatoid arthritis. Many of my most disturbing symptoms were ignored or placed into a new box of "cross-over syndrome." Just what I needed, another diagnosis which meant more drugs. My arthritis wasn't getting any worse but my whole body seemed to be rebelling and I felt that nobody but me was taking it seriously.*

*I began to retreat further into myself until my back was flat against the wall. It was then that I started to push back. I had been hearing people talk about things like naturopathy, acupuncture, and hypnosis, telling me stories about how much they had improved their health and I decided, "to heck with doctors, to heck with the opinion of my family members," I would find the answers another way.*

*I stopped taking my medication and started juicing. I took herbs, antioxidants, fish oil, you name it, I tried it. I went to tai chi three times a week. I learned how to meditate. I saw a hypnotherapist. Instead of listening to doctors, I listened to people who told me that ridding my body of toxins would cure my arthritis. I let my anger and frustration at my doctors, my family, and most of all myself fuel my new quest. I pushed harder and harder to reach the perfect moment when I would be in remission, and I finally got there.*

*For the first time ever I didn't need to rely on an NSAID to get me through the day. My body was free of inflammation and it felt good. The problem was that, although I no longer had a body that was in a constant state of civil war, I was so used to pushing myself I didn't know what it felt like to be comfortable.*

*That was when I decided it would be a perfect time to take off and move to a new town where I didn't know anybody. A small town without any rheumatologists, where I proceeded to become a jack-of-all-trades occupational therapist and a long distance bike rider. I was having great fun except on the days that I felt ill from all the activity and instead of resting, I spent the time angry that my body wasn't performing the way I wanted it to. Gradually, I started to show signs of arthritis again. I would slap a magnet on my knee, wrap it in an ace bandage, and head up the hill. But no herb, magnet, or acupuncturist could stop the fire that had started to burn inside me.*

*My answer to this was to move again. There had to be something wrong with Colorado so I headed to sunny California. In California, the arthritis came back with a vengeance. It didn't take long for me to decide that maybe the doctors were on to something after all, so I said, "Bring on the drugs!" Prednisone, Methotrexate, Plaquenil, Vicodin, Remicaide, Enbrel, Humira, Kineret, Relafen, Vioxx, Minocine, all went into my body within a period of a couple of years and still my knees were as big as grapefruits. I couldn't work, bike ride, hike, even going food shopping took all my energy and that was when a friend was there to carry the groceries for me.*

*There was nothing to do but stop. Stop and look at why I felt the need to chase my tail so much. Humble myself enough to accept help. Learn that I was still me even when I wasn't externally the me I wanted to be. Finally accept myself, arthritis and all.*

*Gradually, I changed my black and white thinking enough to realize that there is a place for doctors and acupuncturists, medicine and juicers. I didn't have to turn my back on one to try the other and if I could figure out a way to use the best of both worlds, I might actually find the balance I was looking for. Deciding to be angry at my doctor because he couldn't think beyond drugs was like trying to get orange juice from a cow, thinking that carrot juice could erase my genetic tendency toward inflamed joints was as useful as believing in the tooth fairy.*

*I finally became a more educated consumer, looking beyond claims when I was contemplating a new treatment. By understanding what complementary and conventional medicine had to offer me I was able to prevent frustration and dashed hopes.*

*The truth is that arthritis is mysterious, complicated, and amorphous. The experience of living with arthritis will challenge you every day. I've learned that in order to meet this challenge head on requires support from a variety of sources. I've found that for me, the medical world has helped enormously to dampen the fire inside my joints and alternative medicine has helped me to rise to the challenge of living with arthritis in a more resilient way. I found that when I stopped pushing so hard to find the answers, I began to listen. My body finally started to calm down and the real healing began.*

*The next chapter isn't going to tell you what works for arthritis or debunk the "quackery" that exists in the world of alternative medicine. There is no one answer for everybody out there and one modality might be appropriate to use at one time and not another. Whether to use alternative healing is a choice in itself, and choosing not to go there at all may be the best answer for some. I will tell you what alternative medicine has to offer, how it is different from conventional medicine, and provide direction for you so you can decide what might be best for you.*

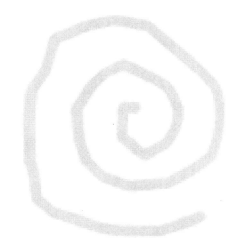

## Chapter Eight:
## Out of the Box, Into the Circle Venturing into Alternative Medicine

> *"Your Current Safe Boundaries Were Once Unknown Frontiers."*
>
> -- *Unknown*

Seventeen billion dollars was spent in the year 2000 on complementary and alternative medicine in the United States. According to the National Center for Complementary and Alternative Medicine, in 2008 thirty-eight percent of adults and twelve percent of children used natural alternatives for healing. To me this is an indirect measure of both the general dissatisfaction with conventional medicine and also a result of the fact that despite all of the amazing advances we've seen in medicine as a whole, our country is getting sicker. Virtually every chronic disease category is on the rise and conventional medicine is scrambling to keep up. Medical doctors are seeing larger numbers of patients because of the pressures from insurance companies and often these patients are sicker. Nearly everyone has some sort of chronic issue, be it rheumatoid arthritis or high blood pressure.

Unfortunately, the conventional medical model isn't set up to treat chronic diseases adequately. Doctors are trained to look for pathologies in bodies, which basically means that a predetermined number, for example a sedimentation rate of under twenty-two for females, has been decided on. If you are out of the normal range you are considered to have a pathological process going on and are diagnosed with a disease. Numbers are good for looking at the general population, but individuals are unique and can vary widely in what is normal for them. This means that medicine is more of an art than a science which creates a tricky situation when doctors are time-pressured and over-worked leaving no time for the artist to come out. The other important consideration in assessing the role of conventional medicine is to realize that doctors are trained mostly as diagnosticians and in prescribing pharmaceutical drugs. This means that, after looking at and finding pathology, they will then turn to prescribing a drug or drugs for the condition.

Hopefully, we all know the goals of taking medication for rheumatoid arthritis; to reduce the inflammation in your joints, decrease pain, and improve quality of life. Many of us have taken a peek at the long list of side effects you get at the pharmacy when you are picking up our medication. What do the side effects mean? Simply put, they mean that by ingesting a synthetic substance that is extremely potent you are taxing your organs, especially the liver, that detoxify the medicine. In addition, drugs most often target more than just your joints which may throw off other systems. This is a necessary evil, part of the cost-benefit that needs to be weighed. We don't take the drug long-term if the costs outweigh the benefits. In fact, some drugs commonly taken for arthritis do have significant drop out rates long-term because of side effects that become unmanageable. The way that physicians deal with this situation is to rotate drugs and luckily these days there are quite a few to choose from before you run out of options. However, this can become a slippery slope, especially when you have a life time in front of you to be taking them.

I'm not in any way trying to undermine or downplay the role of doctors or the importance of medication for serious issues like rheumatoid arthritis. Some of my heroes are my doctors. I'm just trying to point out that there are limits to what they can do in creating a condition for remission in your body. The truth is, health is not just the absence of a pathological process. It is complete physical, mental, and social well-being. Looking at symptom control and reduction of pathology is only the tip of the iceberg when it comes to obtaining and maintaining long-term health. Once you have a chronic disease it is vitally important that you become even more aware of this and invested in addressing all aspects of your health. This is where complementary medicine comes in and where venturing out of the tight box of conventional medicine to explore the ever expanding circle of alternative practices just makes sense. The key is to do so as an educated consumer. This means that you need to understand what you are asking for, understand what you are getting, and be realistic with your expectations of results.

## *Out of the Box*

Understanding what you are asking for means that you understand what complementary medicine is. The simple answer is that complementary medicine is anything that lies outside the scope of conventional medical treatment. The more complex answer is a wide range of healing disciplines, some of which are thousands of years old and others that were discovered yesterday.

What all these disciplines have in common is that they aim to restore balance in order to enhance the body's innate healing capacity. There is sometimes a distinction between complementary practices, which are recognized by the medical field, and alternative, which in general are not considered to have any value by conventional medicine. What is important to remember is that this varies considerably throughout the world. In Germany medical doctors routinely use homeopathy, which in the States is considered alternative; in the Netherlands medical use of saunas is common, another alternative practice here. China brought the value of acupuncture to our attention which now would be considered complementary but not too long ago was alternative. Confused yet?

The bottom line is that our knowledge and acceptance of different approaches is constantly changing. As scientific knowledge grows, so does acceptance. Modern medicine is grounded in the scientific method and therefore any healing discipline or remedy that can't be observed, quantified, and validated by a double blind study will be treated with skepticism. That is the strength of western medicine, but also the source of its rigid thinking and its mechanistic approach.

The approach modern medicine has taken to study something biologically is to break it down into parts and that is why the immune system is studied separately from the nervous system, endocrine system, and so on. Researchers work their whole lives on one portion of one system, say the B cells in the immune system, studying how they function in health and disease. What results from all this intensive study is immense knowledge about the miracle that is our body, along with the tendency to look at things in isolation when an illness manifests itself.

The real problem with organizing our bodies into discrete parts and treating illness as if this was the reality, is that it isn't. The reality is that our bodies are made of layer upon layer of cells that function as individuals supporting a whole. Some cells do double duty for what we call the nervous system and the endocrine system. Some cells change as they grow. What this ultimately means is that the scientific, western medical approach ends up being a two dimensional picture of a three dimensional being. For someone with rheumatoid arthritis it can mean being greeted with a lot of confused looks when you mention that your arthritis gets worse during your menstrual cycle or that you sometimes get hives on your joints.

This has been changing slightly over the course of the past decade as mind/body medicine has been gaining credibility with the established medical community. Doctors, whose belief grows when they can see and quantify something, have found chemicals that actually correlate with emotions. Candace Pert, a researcher who discovered endorphins, termed them the molecules of emotion. These molecules of emotion have been found not only in our brain, but also in our gut, our heart, even our big toe. Molecular tagging, MRI, and other techniques have changed the theory of the mind/body connection into fact. Now that we know this, medicine is trying to figure out what to do with the information and how to alter treatment to fit this new paradigm. Alternative practitioners have known this all along and are already treating the mind/body not as a split but as a continuum. There is no mind separate from the body; the mind is in the body and when an acupuncturist places needles along different points of your body he is aware of this.

Neuroscientists have shown that although humans like to believe that they are logical and analytical, they are actually one big jumble of walking emotions. Most, if not all of our thoughts have an emotion attached to them. Every time we look at another person, hear a sound, or taste a food, both the visual and emotional parts of the brain are activated. It is impossible to separate an experience or a thought from an emotion.

If we come to think of ourselves as one big walking emotion machine we will quickly come to realize how important a positive emotional environment is on our overall health. If you can see that positive physical changes can create improvements in emotions, can you see how the opposite must be true as well? The molecules of emotion are constantly being created and destroyed, and the pathways along which these molecules flow are either sensitized or ignored. If you bathe your body in the molecules of hope, trust, well being, joy, amusement, and ramp down the molecules of fear, anxiety, despair, and helplessness, do you think that your body will see changes? I do, wholeheartedly, and so do the experts in the alternative/complementary medical field.

What complementary medicine has in its favor is that it takes a holistic approach to healing. By looking at the body as a whole it will be easier to see that an imbalance in one place can affect something entirely different. It will be a no-brainer to be aware that what you take into your body and what you assimilate will directly influence your health and well being.  And since the mind and body aren't separate, it will be simple to understand that a calm mind leads to a calm body and vice versa. Complementary medicine is based on the premise that disease is not just a physiological process but a delicate balance of body/mind/spirit, and in some parts of the world this form of medicine has been practiced continuously for thousands of years.   Here in the West we can look back at Hippocrates, the founding father of modern medicine, who in 400 BC recognized the importance of attitude, nutrition, and environment on health and realize we are coming full circle.

## *Exploring Alternative Medicine*

Exploring alternative medicine will consume time, energy, and money. The hope and goal is that the return will be improved energy and reduction of active disease, along with the ability to achieve true healing. When you begin the process of utilizing alternative healers it would behoove you to take a thoughtful approach and begin by doing an assessment. First, ask yourself:

- What do I need at this moment, to help me feel better?

- Can I support my body systems, so they will better tolerate the medication?

- Is there anything I can do to restore balance and enhance healing?

Then consider the following four questions:

- How big is your bank account?

- Whom do you believe?

- How much time and money do you want to spend?

- How much energy do you have to figure it all out?

Let's explore these questions in more depth.

## How big is your bank account?

If it's looking slim, don't panic, you can still do things that will positively affect your health. Low-cost pain relief techniques include heat/cold packs, getting in a quiet place on your back and listening to relaxing music, watching a funny movie, lying in the tub, reading a good book, and good old Ben Gay. I'm sure you can think of more. These are good things to do regularly regardless of your situation. Get into the habit of doing them and keep in mind, improving your emotional state can be as powerful as many physical interventions in improving health and well-being.

## Whom do you believe?

This is where a bit of homework comes in and I'll discuss more specifics about my personal point of view later. The important thing is to look beyond testimonials. I have nothing against them, to me they prove that whatever it is, it has helped at least one person. But does that still mean you have a better chance of getting hit by lightning than improving? With some of the things out there, I'd say yes. When it comes to supplements, I stay away from generic store brands and stick with a few companies that I trust. When it comes to practitioners, talk to them before you go and spend money. Listen to what they are saying and if they tell you they will cure you either hang up or ask them if you would get a refund if they don't. If they seem trustworthy, then ask them how many people with rheumatoid arthritis have they worked with, what they've done, and results they've had. Then, ask how often they want to see you and what they charge. It also helps to ask if they have package deals. Finally, get recommendations from friends. Through word of mouth you can find great people. Many of the most talented healers don't advertise because they don't need to.

## How much time and money do you want to spend?

I consider this a question that has a lot to do with how much you value yourself because I firmly believe in the saying, "Where there is a will there is a way." If you feel you don't have the resources or the time to invest, you can make a decision to be creative in getting what you need. With your available time, take into consideration the *Keeping Joints Strong and Stable* chapter, practice energy conservation, learn to delegate, and plan ahead. If you tell yourself you will find the time, you will. If you do the opposite, eventually you will have plenty of time because your body will flare up and demand it.

As for money, decide to invest in yourself. Avoid getting to the point where you are desperate and vulnerable. Once again, if you put off investing in yourself now eventually you will have to because your body will require it. I know this from personal experience and let me tell you, being desperate and vulnerable is the last place you want to be. You can be creative with this too by being a smart consumer. If massage is something that helps you a lot but the high cost makes it hard to go regularly, consider going to massage therapy schools, the majority of which offer low-cost clinics where you can get a massage at a fraction of the cost. Community adult education classes will offer Tai Chi at a fraction of the cost of a Tai Chi center. Trading services is another idea.

The best way to save money and time is to get the most bang for your buck and this means finding a true healer whom you trust and believe in. This is something I don't have a recipe for, all I can tell you is that it is well worth the effort involved. A true healer will want to know you, will take time for you, will always listen to you, will make you feel completely comfortable, will be with you for the long haul, won't push anything on you that you don't feel comfortable with, and most of all, will bring you results. When you begin looking for an alternative practitioner do your homework about the options available, talk to people you know, see if insurance will pay for any of it, and when you make a choice feel good about it. Don't listen to skeptics who will be glad to tell you what a bunch of malarkey it all is. Let them have their point of view but refuse to buy into it.

The truth is that alternative medicine does help, sometimes a little, sometimes miraculously, and as someone with a chronic issue every little bit helps.

## How much energy do you have to figure it all out?

Like anything worthwhile this will take energy. The key to not getting overwhelmed before you start is to see this endeavor as a process. This means only involving people who will support, not hurt you as you find your way. For me, this has meant that I don't discuss my visit to the acupuncture doctor with my very conventional family members whose eyes glaze over when I start to talk about meridians. Instead, I involve my friends who have made an effort to learn about the benefits of Chinese medicine and who may be using it themselves. This isn't a judgment; it's just a practical way for me to avoid stress and depleting my precious energy. There will be bumps in the road as you begin to delve into alternative medicine, you may have to try out a few people or a few different types of therapy before you find the one that you feel comfortable with. In the end it will be well worth the effort and you will be glad you did.

When you jump out of the box and search for a deeper understanding of your body it is important to keep a few things in mind.

## People will always be biased in favor of their area of expertise.

Like the media, there is no such thing as an unbiased opinion. Go to a surgeon and you'll end up having surgery, go to a chiropractor, and you'll get your back worked on. See a doctor and come home with a prescription, see a naturopath and the prescription will be for a combination of vitamins, herbs, and diet changes. There is absolutely nothing wrong with this, the only red flag would be if any practitioner claims that they have a cure. If they did they'd be a lot richer and too famous to see the likes of you. The undisputed fact is that arthritis is largely a mystery; there are many educated guesses out there but not many absolutes yet. Seeking out the assistance of a naturopathic doctor means you are hiring a consultant for a complex problem. You can use their vast knowledge about their discipline to gather information and then decide the best course of action. If the person you are seeing is telling you something that doesn't sound or feel right to you then trust that feeling, thank them for their time, and move on.

## The results you will see from drugs are often quicker and more dramatic than complementary medicine.

This is because the majority of alternative medicine is aimed at enhancing the body's ability to heal itself. The subtle nature of this process may seem frustrating at times, however you have the consolation that the risk of further morbidity or death is next to nil compared to taking drugs. As I said earlier, pharmaceuticals are largely aimed at symptom management not dealing with the source of the problem. This isn't because doctors don't care about the source of the problem, but because they just don't know. Unfortunately, eradicating symptoms can also be like cutting butter with a chainsaw, hence the commonality of side effects. Until more arthritis drugs are targeted like the new biologics, medical treatments will in general take the chainsaw approach. And, until the true cause or causes of RA are found, doctors will be playing a numbers game with you, giving you the treatments that have been shown to help the most people without the full knowledge about your individual needs.

Alternative healing practices take a wider view and consider disease a byproduct of imbalance in the body. This is why stress is becoming so widely recognized as a factor in the cause of disease; stress is such a strong force in the creation of imbalance. Any disease that a person ends up with is influenced by inherited and acquired weaknesses, but a body in balance will be less likely to manifest disease and if it does, the disease won't be as extreme. Achieving balance does take time, effort, and changing tactics as the body changes. Eventually though, the body will be able to self-correct and fluctuations in a person's health won't be as extreme.

## There are some extremely talented people out there, but you usually have to work to find them.

There is no US News and World Report on the countries best alternative practitioners but there really should be. The most talented practitioners will listen to what you have to say, trust your ability to guide the treatment, and be very willing to tell you that they don't have all the answers. But they will also sincerely try to do everything they know how to in order to get you better. Word of mouth is usually how you find the best people. Start asking around and you'll be surprised at who you may find. Entering a partnership with one or more quality alternative practitioners will enhance your body's ability to tolerate prescription drugs, will improve your overall health, will improve your quality of life, and most importantly, will help you be more in tune with your bodys' needs. And as you become more in tune with your body you will become more confident in your ability to ask and receive what you need, be it from the doctor, chiropractor, masseuse, family member, or yourself. You'll also become much more aware of how your diet, exercise, and lifestyle affects your overall health.

**Skepticism is a good thing, up to a point.** You don't want to eliminate the placebo effect entirely (Just kidding!) Seriously, though people can be very convincing and going back to my first point, they will be biased. Complementary medicine is now seeping into the mainstream which is a good thing. However, people follow the numbers and anytime large amounts of money are being spent in any area more and more people will try to get a piece of the pie. This means that these days you see a Vitamin Cottage in every strip mall, and as someone with arthritis you will be a huge target. Every time you turn around there is another miracle remedy aimed at you. The vast majority of these will be over-hyped and will underperform. In fact, the majority of remedies have very little of the active ingredient on the label insert stats. Some so-called "antioxidants" can be pro-oxidative, meaning they will create more harm than good in your body. If a multivitamin is not food based it really won't do you any good.

The combination of extreme need, vulnerability, and so many people who are convinced that their particular modality is the best can be at times overwhelming. Do you go with the Acupuncture, Massage, Physical Therapy, Chiropractic, Reiki, the latest arthritis supplement, a hot tub, or just good old Ben Gay? Much of complementary healing practices don't have rigid, double-blind studies to prove their efficacy, so knowing what really works can be difficult. If a discipline has been around for a long time, like traditional Chinese medicine or Ayruveda, you can be assured that they will have something to offer because they are time tested.

Where I am most skeptical is in the area of supplements. This is where you'll find a lot of grandiose claims about the newest wonder herb that will cure everything that ails you, with a bunch of hopeful sounding testimonials to back up the claims. The problem with this, besides the obvious one that there is no federal regulation to ensure that there will be anything besides fillers in the capsule you are taking, is that these companies are playing upon our magic pill fantasy. Let me say this once and for all, there is no such thing. No pill will cure an imbalanced body/mind. We may not like to hear this but becoming and staying healthy takes effort. Every day, every hour, every minute. Every thought, action, and decision influences your health and no pill will change this.

## You may have to live with people who judge you for trying non-evidenced based practices.

This is something I have had a lot of practice with and it's still difficult. People have a right to their opinion, but absolutely no right to judge you for trying everything that you feel might help even if there is no hard evidence to support it. Sometimes the intense reaction people have for or against alternative medicine makes me want to start talking about something less controversial like politics or religion. I've been ridiculed, patronized, judged, doubted, condescended to, been told I was "going off the deep end." This from people I love by the way.

When this happens, I try to let go of the hurt it creates in me and I remind myself of what I learned in the book, *Deep Survival.* No one and nothing will break my spirit because there is always one more thing I can do. I can keep going, pick myself up and start over again and again because I will never give up. I believe in my ability to succeed enough to know that I don't need anyone else to believe for me. I know that I have carefully thought through my choices, I have created a plan, a backup plan, and I hold onto both with a gentle grip so I can let go and change course at any time. I stand firm in my decision to look beyond conventional medicine because I know that I need to in order to be a resilient survivor and to live well. I carry this around like internal armor so that I can withstand the force of other people's opinions.

Although I know I would never treat someone this way if the shoe was on the other foot, especially someone I care about, I have to wonder why other people need to and part of me thinks that they are reacting to their own fear about my situation. Sometimes fear and frustration can turn into anger and when this anger has nowhere to go it lands on the person closest to the situation. I know that my loved ones don't want to hurt me, and I know that they do care, and I know how scared I feel at times. This knowledge brings me understanding and forgiveness.

*"Fortitude is necessary, and patience, and courtesy, and modesty, and decorum, and a will in what may for the moment seem to be the worst of worlds, to do one's best"*
*- Marcus Aurelius Meditations*

This leads me to talk about why. Why try to wade through the misinformation, skepticism, judgment, grandiose claims, and unproven treatments when you can just leave your care in the hands of your doctor? Why try if you're unclear about what the result will be? To me this is like asking why get out of bed in the morning if you don't know exactly how your day is going to go. It's asking yourself how you want to experience your life and how you want to view your arthritis. Are you looking to cure or heal, be symptom free or well?

Conventional medicine will help you to eradicate your symptoms; alternative medicine will help you to restore balance. Curing is in the realm of conventional medicine, healing is the aim of alternative practices. Curing your disease will take away unpleasant symptoms so that you can continue to live the life you always have, healing your body will change the way you live, and how you relate to yourself and others. Curing subtracts, healing adds. Curing looks at the body as a biological being.  Healing looks at the body as a manifestation of our thoughts, emotions, biography, and environment.  Curing is recovery from disease. Healing, according to Dr. Lawrence Bendit, is "Basically the result of putting right our wrong relationship to our body, to other people, and... To our own complicated minds with their own emotions and instincts at war with one another and not properly understood by what we call "I" or "Me" The process is one of reorganization, reintegration of things which have come apart."

There is no right or wrong here. If you decide to focus on curing you can still use alternative healers to help you feel more comfortable during the process. You may be restored back to health and be quite content with this. If, however, you are like me and have experienced a continuous fluctuation of a state of cure, disease, cure, disease, you may want to explore a deeper understanding of true healing.

When I first went into remission in my twenties I was so happy about the new things I could do that were impossible before. As a kid I would watch other children sit on their heels and literally have dreams that I could do this when in reality, even kneeling was too painful most of the time. One day a year or so into my remission I sat on my heels and had a moment of total euphoria realizing that a childhood dream had come true. I would go out of my way to squat down and reach for something just because I could. These were small victories for me that I cherished. But I also remember a little voice in my head telling me that it wasn't over yet, my battle with the arthritis was only on hiatus. This voice was actually more of a feeling some would call intuitive. At the time, all I knew was that I pushed it out of my mind whenever it surfaced.

Long before I was consciously aware of the concept of healing versus curing this feeling told me that my remission was temporary because inside I hadn't changed. I was still the person that accepted her body only when it was behaving, that blamed herself whenever the arthritis got worse, that didn't feel safe telling anyone how despairing she really felt at times, that either put on a happy face or hid, that walked around self -flagellating because she didn't measure up, and who felt it was all her fault. I was officially in remission from the arthritis but I was like a war veteran walking around appearing fine but who was having a hard time leaving the battlefield in her head. Until I could put right my wrong relationship to my body I might have been free of arthritis but I was still in chains and because of this I was paralyzed when the arthritis started to stir again inside. For me, alternative healers have enabled me to look beyond my sedimentation rate and begin to see my body for what it truly is, a full human being that wants to be comfortable and relaxed. By looking past the word cure I have been able to heal the wounds that really hurt and in doing so I know that I am finally free.

## *Into the Circle, Exploring Complementary Medicine*

*Physical modalities:*
Tai chi, Yoga, Chi gung, Feldenkrais, Alexander technique

*Passive manipulative modalities:*
Acupuncture, Reiki, Massage, Cranial sacral therapy, Myofascial release, Reflexology

*Biologically based:*
Herbal supplements, Nutriceuticals, Juicing, Fasting, Diet

*Passive non-manipulative:*
Sauna, Hypnosis, Biofeedback

*Energy Therapies:*
Reiki, Chi gung, Therapeutic touch, Energy medicine

*Disciplines:*
Oriental medicine, Naturopathy, Osteopathy, Homeopathy, Ayurvedic medicine, Chiropractic

## *Chapter Eight Worksheets*

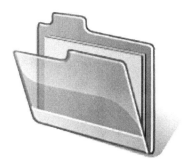

- Questions to Ask Yourself
- Questions to Ask Your Alternative Healer

# QUESTIONS TO ASK YOURSELF

What do I need at this moment, to help me feel better? _____

_____

_____

_____

_____

_____


Can I support my body systems, so they will better tolerate the medication? _____

_____

_____

_____

_____

_____


Is there anything I can do to restore balance and enhance healing?_____

_____

_____

_____

_____

_____


What is my plan? What is my back up plan? _____

_____

_____

_____

_____

_____

_____

_____

**QUESTIONS TO ASK YOUR ALTERNATIVE HEALER:**

*1. Have you treated people with rheumatoid arthritis before? What successes have you seen?*

*2. What is your philosophy of healing?*

*3. What is your education?*

*4. How will you help my body to feel better?*

*5. How will you help me to support my body systems so I can better tolerate my drugs?*

*6. How will you help me restore balance and enhance my healing?*

*BEWARE OF:*

- *THE WORD CURE*
- *PEOPLE WHO ARE COMPLETELY AGAINST CONVENTIONAL MEDICINE*
- *PEOPLE WHO SAY THEY KNOW THE CAUSE OF ARTHRITIS*
- *PEOPLE WHO SAY ARTHRITIS IS CURED BY DIET*
- *PEOPLE WHO WANT YOU TO COMMITMONEY UP FRONT*
- *EXPENSIVE TREATMENTS*

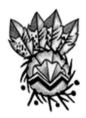

*I've always loved to sleep. To me it's like taking a trip and never knowing where you're going to end up. How endless would life feel if we didn't sleep? How much harder would we push ourselves?*

*I love jumping into bed at the end of the day, getting cozy, maybe reading a good book before drifting off to sleep and waking up eight or nine hours later, ready for the day and remembering some interesting dreams. Unfortunately, this doesn't happen on a regular basis. I remember times in my life when I achieved this almost nightly and I think it must be like the high school football star reflecting on the good old days. These days, sleep for me often feels like walking on a tightrope. If I tip just slightly I can end up falling into a bad sleep pattern. How has sleep become so elusive at times, such a struggle, so inconsistent? How can I reclaim my natural ability to sleep?*

*These questions have spurred me into looking at my past and present sleep habits and trying to decipher which help and which hinder me. By doing this I've learned a few things. I've learned that anxiety and sleep are like oil and water, and worrying at bedtime is one of the worst things you can do to yourself. Other things that can disrupt my sleep; cold feet, noise, light, snoring, getting to bed too late, a mind that doesn't want to shut down, and strangely enough, being over tired.*

*I know arthritis pain is the biggest reason that for me sleep can be so difficult. Pain has always influenced the amount of sleep I need, the fact that it takes me awhile to get to sleep, and how restless I can be when I change positions throughout the night to stay relatively comfortable. The consequences of a poor night's sleep is larger for me than the people in my life who don't have arthritis because it ratchets up the pain and makes me feel like Dr. Jekyll and Mr. Hyde on a Mr. Hyde day.*

*I'm not ashamed to say that I carry a hot water bottle and a pillow for my knees when I travel, along with an assortment of sleep inducing herbs or teas. I'm not afraid to tell people to quiet down when it's my bedtime and I won't take any job that requires me to arrive before the crack of nine a.m. anymore.*

*When it comes to sleep I'm like the princess in The Princess and the Pea. I'm not a prima donna in any other way but this. Sleep is that important to me. It is a requirement for me to be me. So enough about me, let's talk about sleep.*

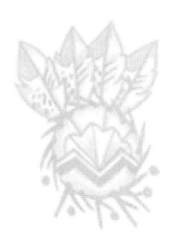

## Chapter Nine:
## HOW TO GET HAPPY ZZZ'S

*"Health is the first muse and sleep is the
condition to produce it."*
                    *-- Ralph Waldo Emerson*

Sleep deprivation is a form of torture and one of the oldest forms at that. The ancient Romans termed it "tormentum vigilae," or waking torture. Sadly, up to 75% of Americans say that they have sleep problems on a regular basis. Even worse, we are getting 20% less sleep than we did a hundred years ago. In 2005, 45 billion prescriptions were written for sleeping pills. It is estimated that approximately five billion dollars a year is spent on sleeping aids. Sleepiness causes more than 100,000 automobile accidents every year, and the infamous disasters of Chernobyl, the Exxon Valdez, Challenger, and Three Mile Island were all attributed to errors in judgment from excessive sleepiness.[53] According to the University of Michigan, we value sleep more than money for happiness and spend one-third of our life sleeping. All of this for an activity scientists still don't agree on why we need.

We may not be able to say why we need sleep, but we do know how we feel when we don't get it. Not only do we feel tired, but our pain tolerance goes down, memory is impaired, reaction time slower, our appetite and cravings increase, as does the tendency to gain weight. How important is sleep? How important is your quality of life? How important is your happiness? Speaking for myself, to paraphrase the MasterCard commercial, "1 cup of coffee, $1.50, good quality sleep, priceless."

In this chapter I will discuss current research about what happens during the night as we sleep, types of sleep issues, the difference between sleep disorders and disordered sleep, why people with arthritis are likely to have sleep issues, and most importantly, what to do about it.

## *Healthy Sleep*

What happens when we sleep? What actually is sleep? Sleep is a very sensitive, regulated process that is a biological need even if the reason for that need is not yet fully known. There are areas of the brain that are devoted only to sleep. Our need for sleep is largely determined by our circadian rhythm which tells us what time of day it is, the number of hours we've been awake, and our cumulative sleep debt, meaning how many hours of sleep we've been getting recently.[54] Sleep involves turning off your conscious perception of the outside world and is characterized by specific, measurable, electrical changes in the brain. It is a complex process involving the endocrine, nervous, and immune systems.

We all have a homeostatic mechanism involving a sleep inducing chemical called adenosine. As we sleep, levels of adenosine drop. The reason that caffeine impairs sleep is that it blocks the receptors for adenosine, keeping levels low which tells the body that we've already gotten the sleep we need.

Our circadian rhythm is governed by a group of nerves in the hypothalamus which are synchronized by light and darkness. As natural light decreases the hormone melatonin is released from the pineal gland and signals to the body that it's time to transition to sleep. Once adenosine and melatonin levels increase, we feel very sleepy and get into bed. This begins the first brainwave shift into a state of calm wakefulness, indicated by a brainwave called an alpha wave. From there, drowsiness yields to stage one sleep and the conscious mind turns off. Stage one is light sleep and easily arousable. In fact, if you wake up from stage one sleep you won't be aware of having slept at all.

Stage two sleep begins very soon after and is characterized by two new sleep specific brain waves called sleep spindles and K complexes. During this stage, muscles alternate between being relaxed and active while body temperature and heart rate decrease. Stages three and four are deep sleep, dominated by a brainwave called delta waves. Stage four sleep is extremely important for cell repair and tissue rebuilding as well as encoding long term memory. In this stage, specific hormones, including human growth hormone, are released to assist with this repair. Growth hormone itself stimulates tissue repair, prevents osteoporosis, increases metabolism, enzyme production and renews almost every cell system in the body. It repairs the damage that has occurred in the body throughout the day. Stage four sleep lasts longer in children and teens than adults and varies between individuals.

The final stage of sleep is what is called rapid eye movement, or REM sleep. It is characterized by fast and desynchronized brain waves, similar to wakefulness. Non- REM and REM sleep cycles alternate every 90 to 110 minutes and occur four to six times per night. As early morning approaches, the hormone cortisol increases in the bloodstream and reaches its peak in the morning.  This hormone gets us ready for the activity of the day.[55]

What I have described is healthy, restful sleep. Unfortunately, what many people actually experience on a regular basis is disordered sleep characterized by disruptions in this pattern. The number one cause for disordered sleep in rheumatoid arthritis is pain.  Other causes include stress, anxiety, parenting, bed partners, hormonal fluctuations, traveling, changes in schedule, diet changes, prescription drugs, and sleep environment. Disordered sleep is different from a sleep disorder in that it is time-limited and usually has an external cause.

## *Take Sleep Seriously*

Sleep disorders are medical conditions, and there are 78 recognized by the American Sleep Disorders Association. They have a variety of causes and are placed into three major groups. Parasomnias include night terrors, sleep walking and talking, sleep paralysis, and bruxism (grinding your teeth). Disorders of excessive daytime sleepiness include conditions like narcolepsy, and are characterized by the tendency to fall asleep unintentionally.[56] Insomnia is the third group and the one that most people with arthritis fall into.

In fact, fifty percent of people with physical disorders suffer from insomnia. Insomnia involves difficulty falling asleep, difficulty staying asleep, early morning awakening, or poor quality, otherwise known as nonrestorative sleep. A person with insomnia can experience one, two, or all three of these issues. Insomnia can be transient, meaning it happens to you every once in awhile for a couple of nights, short term, where it lasts up to three weeks, or chronic, where it lasts more than three weeks.[57]

Sleep issues and rheumatoid arthritis have been studied and specific issues have been identified.  These include difficulty falling asleep, nonrestorative sleep, higher sleep latency (meaning it takes longer to go from full wakefulness to sleep), more daytime sleepiness, more leg movements during sleep, more sleep shifts from one brainwave pattern to another, more mini arousals, more time in alpha brainwave and less time spent in delta brainwave (remember delta brainwave is required for cell repair, tissue rebuilding and storing long term memory). During an arthritis flare-up sleep is even more fragmented. I'm guessing that this is not a surprise to any of you reading this. It's not rocket science to realize that if you're in chronic pain you're likely to have problems with sleep.

But it may be a bit of a surprise to some people that because rheumatoid arthritis is partially an endocrine disease that affects hormones, people with arthritis are at increased risk for insomnia. The mechanisms for this are not completely understood but are related to regulation of melatonin and cortisol, as well as higher levels of inflammatory chemicals called cytokines in the blood. Also, some medications such as anti-inflammatory drugs (steroidal and non steroidal) can decrease melatonin secretion and interfere with the circadian rhythm.[58]

This is a lot of information to throw at anyone all at once so let me ease your mind by telling you that even the worst case of insomnia can be helped. Despite the fact that you already have a few predisposing factors for sleep problems, remember that no matter how frustrating the experience can become, you can rest assured that your body will eventually sleep.

So, what specifically can we do to help the process along? The first thing is to take your sleep problems seriously. Just because sleep issues are commonplace doesn't mean that they aren't a real problem. And given the fact that you are dealing with chronic pain and inflammation to begin with means that you are already going to bed with one strike against you. Pain and inflammation are both sources of body noise which make quality sleep more difficult to obtain. So, no matter how you rate the severity of your sleep issues there is always room for improvement.

How rested do you feel today? How rested have you felt during the past week? Do you know how many hours of sleep you need to feel rested? We all have our own personal sleep number which may go up and down slightly when your body is more or less challenged, but for the most part it stays the same. As I said at the beginning of the chapter mine, is about eight and a half hours. If you have no idea what your sleep number is try to keep a sleep diary for a couple of weeks, or if your schedule allows you to do this, go to sleep at the same time every night without an alarm clock and see when you naturally wake up. Once you start waking up at the same time every morning you will know how many hours you really need. The complicating factor for people with RA is that if we are experiencing nonrestorative sleep, the number of hours isn't as relevant because you still may wake up unrefreshed. This is an issue I'll talk more about later on in the chapter.

What is your history with sleep? I've always been someone who takes awhile to get to sleep. Normal sleep latency, or the time it takes to get to sleep, has never applied to me and when my sleep issues have been at their worst this has served to increase my anxiety around my sleep. The fact is that the sleep-wake system is complex and some people are naturally endowed with a stronger or weaker sleep system.[59] Many people will find that poor sleep runs in their family. If this is true for you, just like any genetic tendency you can use this knowledge to plan ways to work around it.

 Sleep issues can also become chronic when a short bout of insomnia begins to take on a life of its own and lasts well beyond the time that the original issue that caused the insomnia is resolved.[60] If your insomnia has persisted it will behoove you to begin thinking about when your poor sleep began. Was it during an arthritis flare? An especially stressful period in your life? When you had children? A change in diet? A change in your relationship? If you can narrow it down to a time but not an event, begin to ask yourself questions about your life during that time to help you. What was going on in your life when the sleeplessness began? What were you doing, thinking and feeling? Who was around you? Did you change any sleep habits at that time? These questions will help you to identify whether the sleep change was due to stressful thoughts or negative emotions, a change in your circadian rhythm, or a change in your health. Often the real culprit isn't the event that induced sleeplessness, but how you coped with that event. Change your coping skills and your insomnia will change for the better.

For me, insomnia issues were a gradual process that turned into a crisis when I was hit with a number of stressors and then went into a monster flare up. During this time I tried hard to cope with my poor sleep as well as I could, not knowing that I was subtly sabotaging my own efforts. I started becoming very rigid with my sleep routine, forcing myself to adhere to a specific bedtime even if I wasn't completely tired because I was convinced that was the only way I'd get the hours I needed. I went through a period where I self-medicated with Benadryl almost nightly because I was so emotionally distraught. I took herbs to relax my mind and body every night, but managed to condition myself that I needed them to sleep. I was in so much pain I couldn't exercise the way I normally did.

The most harmful thing I did to myself during this time was to begin ruminating about what a poor sleeper I was. I also became an expert worrier about a lot of other things that never seemed to bother me before. As my body continued to scream at me, I used my precious energy to run around in circles trying to fix things and think up new ways to kick myself for some imagined screw up. I was creating tension in a body that was tense already from dealing with high levels of pain. I was stimulating my fight-or-flight response to such an extent that I was altering my sleep system into one that favored arousal over sleep. It took me years to finally change this for the better, and I did this by learning and practicing ways to enhance my ability to sleep.

Do you feel that your lifestyle is conducive to good sleep? If it isn't, is the cause something you have less control over, like being a new parent or a bed partner that snores? When you are going through a period where your lifestyle makes sleep difficult you can focus on getting the core sleep you need and then compensating with naps throughout the day. Core sleep is the amount of sleep your body needs in order to maintain your performance and studies have shown that for most people this is five and a half hours.[61] For people with arthritis it will probably be more but the key is that you can function just fine for prolonged periods of time getting core sleep only and you don't need this sleep to be uninterrupted to be effective for you.

As a new parent, if you are getting three hours here and four hours there, you may be fine. Just remember to check in with your accumulated sleep debt periodically. If you find that you are starting to fall asleep during the day at unexpected times then you have acquired a sleep debt that needs to be addressed somehow. The last thing you need is to fall asleep at the wheel.

Bed partners can be a touchy issue because the reality is that two people sleeping in the same bed will negatively affect each other's sleep.[62] Every time your partner moves in bed you are likely to shift out of deep sleep, and as someone who doesn't reach deep sleep easily to begin with this can have a more adverse effect on you than your partner. This is an issue that you can resolve by talking about it with your partner and problem solving together. One option is to get a larger bed, or sleeping separately during times that you feel your sleep is especially challenged, such as during a flare up or when your pain starts rising.

It's easy to get into habits that sabotage good sleep. Staying up late studying, watching television, staying on the computer, eating large meals late at night, and worrying are all sleep sabotagers. What are your biggest sleep robbers? Changing habits that impede sleep and replacing them with sleep promoting ones is the key to long term change.

Once you begin to understand your own personal sleep print you can begin to change it for the better. Learning the basics of sleep hygiene is the place to start.

## *Creating Sound Sleep*

Here are the basic rules of good sleep habits, otherwise known as sleep hygiene:

**1. *Have a regular bedtime and try to get up at the same time every morning if possible.***

The condition to this rule is that you really shouldn't go to bed unless you feel tired so don't be too strict with yourself, especially if you are already suffering from insomnia. And during a flare getting up a little later may actually help. However, keep in mind that when you get up later you are altering your circadian rhythm and if you do this too much you will be setting yourself up for more sleep problems. On days that you feel the need to stay in bed a bit longer spend some time outside in the morning and get some light exercise to raise your body temperature if you can.

**2. *Establish a bedtime ritual, which allows your body and mind to relax and become drowsy.***
Allowing the body to relax is the key to encouraging sleep. Things that should not be included in this ritual involve activities that require bright lights, which will disrupt your circadian rhythm, sitting in front of a computer, chatting on the phone, or, believe it or not, a very hot bath right before bed. Warm baths are wonderful, but your body temperature needs to drop when drifting into the first stages of sleep so it's better not to take a bath and then hop into bed right away. Better options include light reading, relaxing music, using scented candles or aromatherapy ( Lavender, lemon balm, rose, and sandalwood are all good choices as they have calming effects on the nervous system), drinking herbal tea, and of course, getting into your most cozy pajamas. Use your ability to condition your body to work for you, not against you.

 Having a bedtime ritual will enable your body to unconsciously learn sleep cues by beginning to associate certain behaviors with sleep instead of frustration and arousal. If you can sleep in your living room but not your bedroom, or if you feel tired until your head hits the pillow, you have conditioned yourself for wakefulness and you can turn this around by using new associations. Go through your nightly ritual and see how your body feels. Do some actions relax you and others cause anxiety? Pay attention and create a bed time ritual that works for you. Two pillows, a hot water bottle, or a glass of milk, do whatever it takes to help you feel relaxed. It doesn't matter how strange these rituals may seem (Charles Dickens always had to have his head pointing north). Just keep in mind that if you won't be able to maintain your ritual in other places you may be setting yourself up for transient insomnia when you are in different surroundings.

### 3. *Use food.*

Whenever possible eat light meals at night emphasizing complex carbohydrates and try to have your last meal three hours before you go to sleep. It's best to avoid placing strain on your digestive system at night because that can impede sleep. Light snacks at bedtime, however, are actually fine and can be sleep promoting. The best bedtime snacks have tryptophan in them which boosts serotonin levels, a brain chemical necessary for normal sleep. These include foods such as turkey, bananas, figs, dates, yogurt, honey, milk, tuna, and whole grains such as oats and brown rice. Melatonin is found in cherries which may be something to try before bed as well, especially since they have anti-inflammatory properties too.

Avoid caffeine, alcohol, sugar, cheese, chocolate, bacon, ham, sausage, eggplant, spinach, potatoes, and tomatoes close to bedtime as these foods contain tyramine, an amino acid that can perk up the brain.[63] Eating high protein foods can block the synthesis of tryptophan so if you are eating protein just don't overdo it.  Some vitamins and minerals can help promote sleep as well. The B vitamins, especially B6 can assist sleep by increasing the effectiveness of tryptophan. Calcium has a calming effect on the nervous system as does magnesium. Low levels of magnesium in particular have been shown to lead to shallower sleep and more micro arousals during sleep. Deficiencies of folic acid and copper have both been found to contribute to insomnia so it is wise to either take a food based multivitamin containing these, or else including foods with these essential nutrients especially if you are taking any arthritis medications that deplete them.

The bottom line is that by slightly changing your diet and adding a light, sleep promoting snack at bedtime you will be aiding your body's natural ability to get the rest it needs. Experiment with different foods until you are satisfied with the result. You may find that by keeping a banana by your bed and eating it when you wake up in the night is the best solution or you may find that a glass of milk and toast with honey is the key.

**4.** *Aromatherapy can be a fun and creative way to enhance your sleep.*
The olfactory system is a very primitive and influential sensory system in the brain closely linked to emotions and memory which is why the use of smell can have a profound impact your ability to relax. Essential oils are distilled plant essences that can be used in a variety of ways to help with sleep. A few drops in a warm bath (not hot) In the evening on your pillow, or infused in your bedroom are all good options. Particularly good oils to use include chamomile, lavender (one of the safest and most widely used and also a pain reliever), lemon balm, rose, neroli, sandalwood, cedarwood, and marjoram. Make sure that you use them as directed and heed warnings as they can cause allergic reactions and may not be appropriate for some people.

**5.** *Exercise can also help to promote sleep for a number of reasons.*
Exercise causes your body temperature to rise significantly and then drop a few hours later which will help you to fall asleep and stay asleep as long as you exercise three to six hours before bedtime and no less. Exercise stresses the body physically and in order to compensate for this the brain will increase the amount of deep sleep during the night. This is important for people with RA, since as I said earlier, we don't get as much of this essential type of sleep as other people. More deep sleep during the night will mean that we'll wake up feeling more refreshed. If you exercise outdoors you will enhance your circadian rhythm by exposing yourself to sunlight. This is something to keep in mind when traveling to places in a different time zone.[64]

**6.** *Use the sun.*
Our circadian rhythm is tied to sunlight, another thing we inherited from the days before artificial light. A day spent inside is a day spent in the dark according to our bodies because sunlight is so much more powerful. Using the measurement for light, the luxe, compare a brightly lit room at 500 luxes to the sun at noon, 100,000 luxes, and you'll realize how drastic the difference is. This explains seasonal affective disorder, (when people get depressed during the months with less sunlight), why up to ninety percent of blind people experience insomnia, and why a day spent enjoying the outdoors is a recipe for a great night's sleep. Exposing yourself to sunlight at certain times of the day can help with difficulty

falling asleep (sleep onset) and early morning awakenings. For difficulty falling asleep expose yourself to the morning sun and for waking early go outside in the evening.[65]Also, remember that bright lights late at night will decrease your body's natural melatonin production, so dim the lights an hour before bed.

### 7. Learn to nap.

Scheduling naps into my day has been powerful for me in more than one way. During the time in my life that my insomnia was at its worst, napping was proof to me that my body really could fall asleep. When my arthritis has flared, napping gives me the extra rest my body needs. When insomnia has started to creep into my life, naps help to keep down my sleep debt. And finally, naps keep me more energized and productive longer. When I have a good nap I feel better until I begin to wind down for the day.

As a napper I know I'm in good company. Winston Churchill and Lyndon Johnson were two famous nappers. I also know that I'm on the cutting edge of a new societal trend, one in which some companies now have nap times and nap rooms for their employees. When I take a forty-five minute nap I'm improving my alertness, reaction time, and performance capacity for the next six hours. [66]Napping after being awake for seven hours is a great rule of thumb, one that coincides with siesta time.

I actually tricked myself into learning this skill. A few years ago I was experiencing the worst flare up in my life and literally could not make it through the day without lying down for awhile. I had convinced myself that I couldn't nap because the pain was so bad and sleep had become so elusive. I decided to experiment with relaxation CD's and discovered something called brain wave audio technology. Basically, this is a way to use music and sound frequencies to enhance the production of different brain waves, thereby inducing deep relaxation, sleep, or healing. I began lying down listening to one of the CD's that enhances meditation and found that I was falling asleep. I was amazed and relieved and looked into finding a CD for sleep. I now use this technology as a way to help my body produce more delta brain waves on nights that pain is interrupting my ability to sleep restfully, and during the day to enhance my ability to get into full relaxation. Among sleep experts this may seem like a crutch, but for someone like me it is a lifesaver. And I've finally gotten to the point that I can say without hesitation that I really can nap, with or without my relaxation CD.

**8. *Think about limiting your time in bed.***
This is a common technique that experts use with people who have primary insomnia, or insomnia that isn't linked to a medical condition. Limiting your time in bed will mean that most of those hours will be spent sleeping and this will increase what is called your sleep efficiency. Sleep efficiency is the ratio of your time asleep divided by your time in bed or:

<u>**Time Asleep**</u>
**Time in Bed**

Normal sleepers average ninety percent, people with insomnia, sixty-five percent. If your sleep efficiency is poor it may be time to try spending one hour less in bed. Once you reach a sleep efficiency of eighty-five percent you can add time in bed by fifteen minutes per night as long as you stay at that level of sleep efficiency. What this does is condition your body to associate the bed with sleep as well as increase your body's desire for sleep.[67] In order for your body to get the rest it needs and keep pain levels down you may combine this with adding time in the day for napping or relaxation.

**9. *Here's another excuse to learn to manage your stress levels.***
Stress can affect sleep in many ways. We've all experienced a racing mind when our bodies are tired and know how frustrating that can be. And those of us who've had problems with insomnia also know too well that not sleeping can make the very act of going to sleep stressful. This can become another viscous cycle, because, as I said earlier, the longer sleeplessness occurs the more stressed you feel around sleep. Stress management, specifically practicing relaxation and/or meditation and replacing negative sleep thoughts have been shown to be just as effective as sleep medication in reducing insomnia.[68]

Refer to the chapter, *What's Stress Got To Do With It?* and start to practice some of the techniques I talked about. A good place to start is simple deep breathing. Deep breathing will automatically turn off the stress response and begin to relax your body. Deep breathing with a positive thought will increase that effect. Take a deep breath and say, "I sleep soundly and deeply," "I am relaxed and calm." Now how do you feel? Do this throughout the day and you will begin to notice subtle changes in your body and mind. When you find yourself thinking something negative about your sleep use the cognitive restructuring technique I described in the chapter on stress and learn to turn those thoughts around. Use your new thoughts and combine them with deep breathing to change negative thinking into a way to heal yourself.

**10. *Think about experimenting with our herbal pharmacopeia.***
Herbs are an effective alternative to sleep medications which can have a number of drawbacks for long term use. Sleep medications may cause a hangover effect in the morning, can cause rebound insomnia when you stop taking them, many can be addictive, and disrupt our body's natural sleep rhythms. The most disheartening fact is they can lose their effectiveness over time.

There are a number of very good herbal sleep formulas on the market today and I recommend experimenting with them if you are having difficulty with your sleep. Some herbs that are well known and widely used sedatives are valerian, hops, passionflower, chamomile, lemon balm, kava, catnip, and skullcap. Catnip, hops, skullcap, and chamomile are also pain relievers sometimes used by herbalists for rheumatism so there is an added benefit to using these herbs. Three other supplements worth mentioning are 5 HTP, tryptophan and melatonin. 5HTP is the precursor to tryptophan, an amino acid which helps to make serotonin, a brain chemical that induces sleep. Melatonin, as I mentioned earlier, is a hormone produced by the pineal gland involved with our circadian rhythm and it tells our brain that it is night time. Supplementing with melatonin can be effective for inducing sleep. Since melatonin is a hormone it should be used with caution and not for a long period of time. One interesting fact is that steroids decrease your production of melatonin, perhaps one of the reasons a side effect of these drugs is insomnia.

### 11. *Look around your bedroom, how conducive to sleep is it?*
The ideal bedroom would be dark with the shades down, quiet, uncluttered and cool. A comfortable mattress is important, as is a good pillow. There are no hard and fast rules around this, only that you are comfortable in bed and can stay that way for at least most of the night. In the past I've used egg crate mattresses and feather beds to provide my joints some extra cushioning and I swear by my cervical pillow that I got through a chiropractor. I also use a knee pillow to help with knee and hip pain. If you find that you are waking up with considerable joint pain you may want to think about ways to alleviate your pain there. The other issue for people with challenged sleep is noise. If outside or inside noise is a problem for you think about purchasing earplugs, (I've found that the silicon ones are the best, they can be molded to fit into any ear), or using white noise from a fan to block unwanted noise outside the bedroom.

And last but not least, keep computers, televisions, and anything else that would serve to stimulate your senses out of the bedroom.

### 12. *Stop looking at the clock.*
I guarantee it won't help you to go to sleep and will amp up any anxiety you may be feeling about the fact that you are still awake.

### 13. *The last thing anyone should do is try to sleep.*
Sleep is something you allow yourself to do, not force yourself to do. This means that you should go to sleep when you are tired. If you find yourself becoming rigid about your bed time because you are determined to get enough sleep, start throwing the clock out window. Don't pay attention to the time, pay attention to your body. When your body begins to show signs of fatigue that is your cue to start turning down the lights and begin your nighttime rituals. When you find yourself trying to sleep while in bed, distract your mind and think about something pleasant but not stimulating, the proverbial counting sheep technique. For me, reading before bed helps me to do this As I turn out the light I find myself thinking about my book instead of whether I'm sleeping.

**14. *Be pro-active about your pain control techniques when pain becomes a hindrance to sleep.***

Start to place speed bumps in your day, using that slow time to assess your pain level and do things to bring that level down. Don't wait until bedtime because pain is stimulating to your body and it will take awhile for your body to wind down once your pain has decreased.

**15. *When you have to, use sleep medications judiciously.***

The long-term use of sleep medications is controversial among sleep experts but most do agree that in the short term sleep medications can have a place in the treatment of insomnia. Either over the counter or prescription sleep medications can be used when your schedule has been disrupted to get you through a time-limited, stressful event or to keep pain levels down during a bout of transient insomnia. Talk to your doctor about the most appropriate option for your needs. Given the side effects of sleep medications I talked about earlier it's important to know that they are not addictive and there is absolutely nothing wrong with taking them for awhile. The only danger is emotional dependence when you begin to become convinced that you need the sleeping pill in order to sleep. Using drugs to help you through sleep crises can help you keep your pain levels down and manage your stress with more ease. Once you manage to take away enough sleep distracters you can wean yourself off the medications.

**16. *Have a plan for handling short periods where you know your sleep will be disrupted.***

Traveling, staying with relatives or friends, overdoing it, and hormonal shifts due to your menstrual cycle are all examples of things that you can anticipate and plan for. The key is to do so without going into negative sleep thoughts and planning in your head that you will sleep poorly at these times. Make the adjustments that you need and let it go.

**17. *Make no bones about the fact that as a person with arthritis you need more sleep than people without your challenge.***

It is what it is. This is something you don't have control over so there is no use in spending any mental energy on it.

### 18. *Limit or eliminate alcohol, smoking, and caffeine.*
Alcohol may help you to fall asleep but it impairs deep sleep and makes sleep more fragmented. Caffeine and nicotine are both stimulants.

### 19. *If you feel that nonrestorative sleep is an issue for you, address it sooner rather than later.*
Remember, nonrestorative sleep is characterized by waking up after a full night's sleep and feeling unrefreshed. It is now known more widely in the medical community that fibromyalgia, chronic fatigue syndrome, and rheumatoid arthritis can all involve sleep cycles that are called alpha-delta sleep, or alpha intrusion. This is when both alpha and delta brainwaves are happening at the same time, something that isn't normal and isn't healthy because your brain is getting the signal that it is both awake and asleep and the body isn't getting the deep sleep it needs for recovery. If you feel that you are suffering from nonrestorative sleep, talk to your doctor. Then start an exercise program if you haven't already; there is evidence that exercise helps to alleviate nonrestorative sleep. The other two things that can help are low doses of Elavil, and learning to handle stress in a better way.[69]

### 20. *Uncover any other medical issues that may be contributing to your insomnia and take them to the experts.*
If you feel there may be something else contributing to your sleep issues go to a sleep clinic. They are a lot easier to find these days and a lot better at what they do. Sleep apnea, a condition that causes you to stop breathing during your sleep is very common (up to forty percent of the population) and very disruptive to your sleep and your health.[70] It is also very treatable. A sleep clinic will be able to uncover sleep apnea and any other elusive conditions that may be contributing to your poor quality sleep.

### 21. *And, finally, most importantly, learn what works for you.*
I know people that sleep best with music playing and others who like to bundle up under five blankets. Despite what I've told you or what you read from the experts, you know your own body best. If you feel comfortable doing something that defies all logical reasoning, go for it as

long as you know this is enhancing your sleep. As I said earlier, part of sleep is a conditioned response and if your body is conditioned to drink chocolate milk at bedtime and you feel this helps there is no reason to stop. As much as I've heard that the bedroom should only be used for sleep and sex, it's not going to stop me from reading a bit in bed before going to sleep every night. It's been my ritual since I was a kid, it doesn't affect my ability to get to sleep at night, and I'm not going to change this. The only caveat to this is activities that disrupt your body rhythms. If you are watching television in a brightly lit room before bed you may want to alter this behavior a bit by turning out the lights and see what happens.

Sleep can be your friend, not your enemy. Know that despite any issues you have that challenge your ability to sleep, restful, quality sleep is not out of your grasp. Make this a priority and you'll be amazed at the changes you will see.

# *Chapter Nine Worksheets*

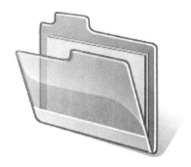

- Sleep Log
- Indentifying My Sleep Detractors
- Changing Sleep thoughts

# SLEEP LOG

Time I went to bed: _____

Approximate time it took me to fall asleep: _____

How many times did I awaken during the night? _____

Pain level at bedtime: _____

Pain level in the morning: _____

Time I got out of bed: _____

Number of hours I slept: _____


On a scale of one to ten how was my sleep quality last night? _____

On a scale of one to ten how refreshed did I feel this morning? _____


Did I take any herbs or medicines to help me sleep? They are: _____

_____

_____

_____

_____


Did I nap, practice relaxation, pain management techniques or stress management techniques yesterday? They were: _____

_____

_____

_____

_____


Is there anything else that I feel affected my sleep positively or negatively last night?

_____

_____

_____

_____

# IDENTIFYING MY SLEEP DETRACTORS

Do I feel anxious at the thought of going to bed? What are my thoughts around this?

_____
_____
_____

Do I often find that my mind is racing when I lie in bed? What are my racing thoughts?

_____
_____
_____

Do I try to fall asleep, or do I just let it happen? _____

_____
_____

Is my sleep easily disrupted when I'm in a different setting or if I have a big day the next day and feel that I need a good night's rest? _____

_____
_____
_____

Does my pain affect my sleep, does my sleep affect pain? _____

_____
_____

## CHANGING SLEEP BEHAVIORS

List at least three things to take away or change In order to achieve better sleep. They can be thoughts, foods, behaviors, items, etc. _____

_____
_____
_____
_____

List at least three things to add In order to achieve better sleep. _____

_____
_____
_____
_____

## CHANGING SLEEP THOUGHTS

| My Sleep Defeating Thoughts: | Reframed Thoughts That Are More Positive And Realistic: |
|---|---|
| "I always have a hard time getting enough sleep." | "For most of my life sleep hasn't been a problem for me. My body knows what to do." |
| "I'm going to be tired tomorrow and I need to feel good." | "As long as I get my core sleep, I'll be able to function just fine." |
| "Darn it, I'm still awake!" | "I always fall asleep sooner or later. Let me use this time to practice breathing and thinking relaxing thoughts." |

## Add yours here:

| My Sleep Defeating Thoughts: | Reframed Thoughts That Are More Positive And Realistic: |
|---|---|
| | |
| | |
| | |

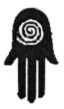

*Language is limited in its ability to express human emotions, especially deep joy and deep pain. When it comes to the expression of the many emotions of rheumatoid arthritis, the limitations of language become abundantly clear and it can be easy to withdraw instead of trying to express your feelings and needs.*

*For much of my life I used the "need to know rule." If another person needed to know something about the arthritis, I'd tell them. If they didn't, I wouldn't mention it. This always seemed to work well for acquaintances and coworkers but with loved ones it often created tension. The tension came from my feeling that those closest to me should care enough to think of my needs without having to admit that I had any. But, because I never spoke up I always ended up accommodating to their needs instead. This usually resulted in exhaustion and disappointment on my end, and frustration on theirs. What I didn't think through for much of my life was that in essence, I was getting upset because my loved ones weren't mind readers. Even worse, if I did speak up I ended up feeling a sense of failure because I was giving a voice to the part of me that I didn't want to own up to, my arthritis. This inevitably ended up as a no-win situation and a recipe for depression and isolation.*

*Using the "need to know rule" for so long made me suffer from not only the physical challenges that arthritis brought but from having to go through life without being able to share with anyone the experiences and challenges that the arthritis brought to me. I suffered alone.*

*Until, in my early twenties I began to take baby steps with a few people I trusted. I found that when I opened up about my life we became closer. I also discovered that the tough circumstances I've handled gave me a level of compassion and a capacity for understanding that few people share. By opening up about my life I am able to show others a profound empathy for whatever hardships they are experiencing. Most importantly though, learning how to communicate well has helped me to grow closer to my family, and transcend the no-win situation of isolation that I lived with for so long.*

## Chapter Ten:
No Man is an Island

*"I think the greatest thing in the world is to believe in people."*
*-- John Galsworth 1867-1933*

"I don't underestimate the contribution of my friends and family members, but the reality is that I faced deafness by myself. And, of course, that's the way it must be in the end. It's how you deal with personal crisis that determines the outcome. Others can offer emotional support, love, sensitivity. But it is up to you to change how you feel."

Reading the experiences of Kiril Sokoloff in his book *Personal Transformation,* who became deaf as an adult is a sharp reminder that having a chronic health issue is a very lonely experience. Regardless of the specific issue or disability, feelings of isolation are part of every day. You will no longer be able to be completely independent, only the most sensitive of people can begin to understand your needs, and asking for what you need can be a quandary. When do you speak up and when do you let the people around you continue to be unaware of what you are going through?

Here's Kiril again

> *"...a professor of history, is giving a lecture. She shows us a slide presentation of ancient art. The overhead light is on at the beginning of the presentation, but after a few minutes her husband turns the lights off. Without lights, I can no longer comprehend her lecture, but the twenty people in the room see the intricate beauty of the slides more clearly. The dilemma? Do nothing, miss the lecture, enjoy the slide show, and be happy that everyone has a clear view of this beautiful, ancient art? Or to make a fuss and turn the lights back on? Of course, I choose to remain silent, as I have a thousand times, when the people turn down the lights, turn up the music, take me to noisy restaurants, and talk at the same time, interrupting each other constantly."*

I've been in a similar circumstance thousands of times as well. It's not a question of whether I'll understand the conversation, but of how much the activity will increase my pain or drain my energy. In both cases though the quality of the experience is diminished. And worse, if I call attention to my needs I risk taking away from the experience of everyone else around me.

## *Opening Up*

So how do you go about communicating your feelings and needs with regard to your arthritis? Who do you choose to explain your circumstance to? How long a learning curve do you allow those around you before you decide that the filter of their experience will limit their ability to understand yours?

The hard thing about chronic disease is that it's chronic. I state the obvious to emphasize how important it is to understand how relationship dynamics change when a person develops a chronic health issue. It is something you just can't fully share. But there is a big difference between feeling lonely and being alone. You may have to face your arthritis alone but you don't have to be lonely while you do it. You are alone because you are experiencing something that is unique and can never be fully understood by those around you. But loneliness comes only when you feel destitute of sympathetic companionship.

The challenge is to cultivate companionship even when you are feeling at your lowest, which is exactly when you need it most. This is a courageous act. The key to opening the door to relationships that feel safe, supportive and comforting is to know what you need to feel good and be able to tell this to people you love without falling into self- blame, defensiveness, passive-aggressiveness, or anything else that will further the divide between you and those around you. This can be really tough, communication is hard enough, but like I said it's more than worth the effort it takes to get there.

## *Finding Self-Worth*

As with most things, improving your relationship with others begins with looking in the mirror. The physical scars of rheumatoid arthritis don't hold a candle to the daily hits to your self esteem and the emotional scars that are created. How to feel good about yourself when some days it hurts to eat, when the grass in your yard grows wild because it hurts too much to turn on the mower, when you realize that someone else must have put gas in the car before you because the gas cap is on so tight you can't unscrew it, when you end up letting the faucet drip because there is no way you are going to be physically able to fix it? To feel good about yourself at times like these takes some creativity, but it's something that you have to do if you do nothing else for yourself ever. And it may be something that you'll need to do again and again, because the arthritis will inevitably continue to humble you.

**When my self-esteem takes a hit:**

- I remember that this may be my situation now, but this too shall pass.

- I do something for someone else in need, and this reminds me that I have a lot to offer.

- I remind myself that I am so much more than the arthritis.

- I try to see the humor in the situation.

- I remember that if I keep trying and do my best every day, I am doing as much as anyone on the planet.

And eventually I find that my self-worth has come back to me. Until it does I won't be able to have a loving relationship with anyone else. Lack of self worth isolates, self respect unites.

## *The Healing Sequence*

Once you have been able to reclaim your self-worth the next step is to begin to move towards creating and strengthening mutually supportive relationships with your loved ones. In the book, *Communication Skills That Heal, a practical approach to a new professionalism in medicine*, Barry Bub, MD describes a healing sequence which looks like this:

**Trauma → Losses → Suffering → Lamenting → Listening → Healing**
Notice that healing takes listening and listening usually involves another person. Notice also that the first two things in this sequence happen to you and the last four are things that you take an active part in. That means that in order to get to healing you need to start with your experience with suffering and in order to do this you need to know where your suffering is coming from. As Victor Frankl said, "Emotion, which is

291

suffering, ceases to be suffering when we form a clear and precise picture of it." Usually, an uncomfortable emotion is the first sign to you that something is amiss. If you start with identifying your emotional reaction you can work backwards to identify the losses that led to your suffering. Let's think of a few losses that most of us can identify with.

- The loss of feeling comfortable in your body

- The loss of roles ( provider, athlete, worker)

- The loss of independence

- The loss of self-esteem

- The loss of freedom

Now some emotions that can happen as a result of feeling those losses;

| Frustration | Fear | Grief |
|---|---|---|
| Helplessness | Anxiety | Loneliness |
| Distress | Sadness | Anger |
| Doubt | Confusion | Hopelessness |

I feel grief because I can't do the things I used to, I feel fear because I can no longer provide the way I used to, I feel helplessness because I've lost my self-esteem. And then we are led toward our expression of these feelings, our lament. Lamenting is a term that means, "An expression of suffering, a crying out of pain- physical, emotional, and spiritual"[71] What you express to those around you, your lament, is also the place that strength in relationships is born.

For much of my life I didn't express my feelings around the arthritis. I told myself, "No one can do anything to take the pain away, so why mention it." I said, "I don't want to show my weakness. " "People don't really want to know anyway." "Who wants to be around a complainer."

I used the need to know rule and I ended up alone in my despair. What is important t remember is that an unexpressed lament will create more trauma, loss, and suffering and will serve to isolate you further from those you love. It's also important to remember that by not speaking up you are reinforcing to yourself that your situation is hopeless. Hope lies in reaching out to others, by becoming engaged.

## *Effective Communication*

We all have different communication styles, and we all will fall into bad communication habits when we are feeling vulnerable. Some people have no problem talking about their complaints to anyone that will listen, others, like me, shut down. What I have in common with chronic complainers is that I'm not getting what I need from those around me. In both cases communication is being thwarted in some way.

If you find that when you express your lament you aren't getting the response you need it's time to work on your communication style. Think about times when you've not felt cared about, heard, validated, supported, understood, appreciated, and the emotions you felt as a result: perhaps hurt, anger, remorse, fear, anxiety, or resentment. Think about how you respond when a loved one treats you in a way that denies your needs. Do you become defensive, do you become mute, do you attack them, do you blame yourself, do you resort to passive aggressive behavior, do you shift all the blame to them, do you become hopeless? Think of a situation that led to emotional tension or miscommunication in your life recently. Think about how you handled it and the result. Did it resolve well or did it create more friction for you?

The reason we communicate, the purpose for communication, is to express feelings or a message with the intent to receive feedback and validation. The best way to do this is to be clear about your intentions and then to effectively get your message across the way you mean it, both verbally and non-verbally. Your statements should match your intentions. Do you want to receive information, analysis, advice, understanding, reassurance, assistance? Each of these intentions would necessitate a different type of communication.

Let's clarify this with an example.

You are having a bad pain day on a holiday weekend. You and your family have plans to attend a few social engagements where people will be playing fun games that, without pain, you would love to be doing. Everyone is happy and excited; they all have had a good night's rest because they got to sleep in and you spent the night tossing and turning in pain. Here are your options:

1.  Suck it up and attend all your functions, put a smile on your face and don't let anyone know how you are feeling.

2.  Wake up grumpy and stay that way, that is how you feel after all and no one can blame you for it. If they had your pain they would feel grumpy too. Your family and friends will just have to deal with it.

3.  Take a deep breath and explain to your family, "I am in more pain today and it started last night. I was really looking forward to this weekend, I love being with everybody but right now my pain is hampering my enthusiasm. I feel like I have the flu and a sprained ankle at the same time. I'm also upset because I love softball and today I feel too much pain to play. So, I'm going to need help getting things ready for our barbeque and I will also need a nap. I may need to leave early so I can get enough rest for the activities tomorrow. Who knows, maybe if I take care of myself today, things will look better in the morning"

Which scenario have you chosen in the past? Which would you choose today? Which scenario would make you feel engaged if you were on the other end of it?

The first scenario is a passive response, it implies that your needs aren't as important as those of the people around you. Eventually this response will backfire because you will either feel so bad you won't be able to function at all or you will begin to feel resentful that those around you are so blissfully unaware of your situation and eventually you may end up in scenario two. In scenario two, you are sublimating your true feelings and projecting them out to those around you. Because you aren't getting what you need, you unconsciously want those around you to feel as miserable as you do so you let your anger permeate the house. Most of the time when you are in this state of mind you are denying your real emotions around the situation and substituting anger, which is a common distraction technique. The third scenario is an example of effective communication. In this scenario you've pinpointed how you feel (disappointed), identified your lament (not feeling up to participating in something you've looked forward to doing) and expressed your needs (a nap, leaving early, extra help, and rest.) The people hearing this will be very clear and will be able to empathize a lot better with your situation and you will feel a lot more validated in your experience.

I know that love may make the world go round but everyone wants to be understood. Understanding is part of love and communicating well is the first step to mutual understanding. Being able to communicate well when you have a chronic health issue is an act of bravery. It takes real guts because you will end up communicating feelings that aren't fun and opening up makes you vulnerable. Acknowledging your limitations make them real.

 For much of my life I know that, although I was justifying my silence by telling myself that no one could do anything to take the arthritis away, part of me thought that not mentioning it would make it not real. Yes, that is magical thinking I know, but it can be a powerful way to cope for awhile. Like an unexpressed lament, eventually this kind of thinking will do you and those around you a disservice because you aren't being truthful. Good communication and full understanding requires the truth. The other part to this is the vulnerability that comes with opening up. What if you don't get the response you need or hope for? What if the person you are communicating with feeds on your negative emotions and creates more fear? This is when you focus on listening well and standing up for yourself, knowing that in doing so you are giving the other person an opportunity to grow.

## *Listening Well*

Listening well involves listening without judgment and with an uncluttered mind. Listening well involves focusing on what the other person is saying, not what you want to say back. Active listening will give you the opportunity to allow the other person to open up as well. By not focusing on getting your point across but instead focusing on what the other person is trying to say, you will be able to really hear.[72] Listening well can de-escalate strong emotions and give you both more time to understand what the other person is feeling. In the book, *Managing Pain Before It Manages You*, by Margaret Claudhill, a simple technique to do this is described. Use the phrase,

"You sound _____ about _____."

Let's go back to the example and suppose after explaining yourself in scenario three your spouse says, "I don't know why you don't just take a Tylenol, you are so stubborn. If you just took a Tylenol you'd be able to sleep and you wouldn't be so cranky"

Ouch, I know, but let's keep going. Take a deep breath and say, "You sound angry about my deciding not to take drugs every time I feel more pain."

"At least the drugs can take the pain away temporarily."

"You sound certain that Tylenol will take away my pain enough to sleep well."

"I'm just so upset that this is part of your life and I don't feel like there's anything I can do to take it away. You shouldn't have to suffer so much."

"I totally agree, I shouldn't! I get sad too that this is what I deal, with but my experience has been that when the pain gets this bad Tylenol won't touch it enough to allow me to push through with my plans. You don't have to feel bad that there isn't anything you can do to take it away; even the best minds in the world who devote their life to curing this disease haven't come up with anything yet. I think we are both doing the best we can given the circumstance."

"I know, you have such a great attitude. We'll do something really fun when you start to feel better."

This conversation taught you that your spouse feels helpless to do anything and really wants to help which is why he/she told you to take Tylenol. Your spouse feels upset for you but unfortunately projected his/her own feelings of upset onto you. The potential for hurt feelings is huge here, but by using this simple technique you quickly were able to get to the core of the real issue and diffuse upset feelings. At the end your angry spouse complimented you and both parties began to feel closer. The other great thing is that you were able to clarify where feelings were actually being directed, not at you but at the situation, so you didn't have to take it personally. What seemed like a personal attack was actually your spouse's own lament, an expression of his/her suffering around the situation. Because you were able to listen you were able to begin to heal.

## Active Listening

Sometimes the person you are talking to will feed on your fears and end up creating more anxiety. What would happen if your mother called on this holiday weekend and hearing how you feel, said, "Nothing seems to be working for you, your arthritis is getting worse." This may be an underlying fear lurking around in your head and immediately you begin to feel even worse than you did before. What if every time you called your Mom, or vice-versa, when you were feeling bad the conversation went this way?

We all have people in our lives that feed on our fear. When this person is a close loved one, communication can quickly shut down, consciously or unconsciously. Who wants to talk to someone that will make them feel worse? This kind of person will tap into your own negative, distorted thoughts very quickly and instead of escalating you into anger, will sink you into depression or despair. The way to turn this dynamic around is by combining active listening and redirecting the irrational beliefs that you and the other person fall into toward more realistic and healthy thoughts and behaviors.

"Nothing seems to be working for you. Your arthritis is getting worse"

"You sound depressed about the fact that I'm having a bad day. Is it really true that my having a bad day means that my arthritis is getting worse?"

"No, I know that arthritis has its ups and downs, it just seems like whenever we talk you are feeling bad. Your life is so hard."

"I'm sorry it seems that way to you. I sometimes feel this way too, and when I do I try to look at the situation in a different way."

"You really are amazing at all you've accomplished and are able to do. You seem to find the most creative ways to handle your pain."

"Thanks Mom, that's nice of you to say. I'll try to call you on days that I feel good so you can be a part of the fun times. Because you're my Mom you bear the brunt of the times I feel bad. Sometimes I just need someone to listen and a bit of reassurance and I always seem to turn to you for that."

This conversation was very productive in many ways. Not only did you uncover your Mom's distorted, all or nothing thinking around the ups and downs of arthritis, you gave her a way of reexamining those thoughts. You also uncovered a problem; you rely a lot on your Mom for emotional support, and made a decision to help with it which is to call her when you are feeling good so she can be a part of your joy not just your pain.

Changing negative dynamics can be difficult, especially with family or friends with whom you have a long history. Just remember, those are the people you use to learn more about yourself. Watch what buttons they push and you will continue to grow despite their negativity. Watch their fears and you will better understand yours. By being persistent in your communication with them, you will be able to unravel your unhealthy dynamics, which you both contribute to, and strengthen your relationship. As I said earlier, good communication involves speaking the truth, your truth, and listening to the truth of the person you are communicating with.

The other part to this is to be easy on yourself when you don't do it well; when you resort to your automatic response whether it is to go mute and retreat or to go on the offensive and attack. It's unrealistic to think that you can make a decision to change your communication style and then be 100% perfect at it from then on. You're not always going to remain calm, unhurt, and self-assured with every interaction and there will be some people who will be harder to communicate with than others. When you revert back to these self-protective behaviors, give yourself a break, and later on reflect back on the circumstance to help you uncover why you felt so vulnerable. You can always keep learning about yourself as long as you keep trying.

## *Circle of Support*

We all have a limited capacity for understanding. We see the world through the filter of our own experience and some people have a limited capacity to empathize with yours. That's okay, if I challenge myself I know it would take a lot of work for me to fully empathize with someone who lives in a world through the filter of schizophrenia. It makes sense that someone who has never experienced pain will have a difficult time understanding the experience of mine. Even the most well-meaning of people will be limited in their ability to provide you with all that you need from them emotionally. Once you understand this you will be able to see that by cultivating a core group of people who can support you in all the ways you need, you will know who to recruit for help at any given time. I know that sometimes I need to problem solve through a difficult decision that the arthritis has presented to me, other times I need to express my fear to someone who will just listen. At times I need a bit of hope, and every once in awhile I just need my best friend to tell me how great I am.

## *Cultivating Empathy*

Understanding the concept of limited capacity doesn't have to be an excuse for it. Empathy can always be deepened, you just have to have the will and desire for it. Empathy involves increasing your understanding of the other person's experience by shifting your perspective in a non-judgmental way and opening yourself up to their reality. Empathy and compassion are similar. Empathy means, "The action of understanding, being aware of, being sensitive to, and vicariously experiencing the feelings, thoughts and experience of another." Compassion means, "The sympathetic consciousness of other's distress together with a desire to alleviate it."

You need to have empathy in order to feel compassion and compassion is necessary to heal yourself and others. The desire for increased empathy is the desire to heal.

*Compassion for myself is the greatest healer of all*
*-Unknown*

There are many ways you can increase your empathy. You can try to literally put yourself in the other person's shoes by simulating their experience. If I were to increase my empathy for someone who has suffered a stroke I could tape one arm to my side and wear glasses that block some of my visual field.  Although I'd know that in a few hours I'd be able to return to my life, at least I'd be able to get a small taste of the other person's experience.

## Here's another empathy skill training exercise adapted from the Harvard medical School Mind/Body Institute:

1.  Find a partner
2.  One partner will relate a stressful event from his or her life.
3.  As you relate this experience, **don't** name the feelings associated with it.
4.  Take a minute and write down the feelings that were experienced during this event. Have your partner list the feelings he or she

believed you experienced based upon your words and body language.
5. Compare lists and discuss.
6. Switch roles.

Another idea to try is to call a friend and practice. Ask them how they are doing and really listen. Paraphrase what they tell you and reflect back to them what they are saying to you. Remember that most communication involves an intention. What are they intending to convey? What do they need from you, problem solving, advice, reassurance, support? Can you provide that for them? Is there a way you can relate to their situation in any way? Cultivating empathy toward others will not only help you feel better about yourself, but will also help others learn empathy through you.

When does your ability to empathize get challenged? Make a list of situations or circumstances that are difficult for you to empathize with. This will help you to uncover your own biases and see where power struggles come from. Power struggles emerge when one person lacks empathy and tries to mold the other person into the framework of their own experience. Going back to the example of the conversation with your spouse, the person telling you to, "just take Tylenol," hasn't taken the time to put themselves in your place enough to realize that they wouldn't be able to know what will take your pain away. By the end of the conversation understanding was improved on both sides and empathy was starting to be created.

As Steven Covey says in his book, *Seven Habits of Highly Effective People:* "Seek first to understand, and then to be understood." Problems won't be solved until you can hear and understand them fully and this is true for problems with relationships as well. If you can approach a problem in a relationship and think win-win, another Steven Covey concept, you will be able to shift your perspective and in doing so, increase your empathy. Assume that the person you are conflicted with wants to improve the situation as much as you do and go from there. Why are they reacting the way they are? Try to avoid making global assumptions about the other person such as, "They always see the worst in every situation," or, "They always think they know what's best." If you avoid accusations, hostile, or sarcastic remarks you will find that the other person will begin to go there less frequently as well. If you value your own truth and value theirs just as much, you will begin to see their side and eventually come to be on the same side, both working toward the same goal, an improved relationship.

Standing up for myself has given others around me the opportunity to grow. The times in my life when I have taken the time to think about a challenging situation with my loved ones, examined my emotions around it, and then taken the opportunity to talk to them about my experience and how I would like things to change, they inevitably have. Maybe not that day, or even that year, but eventually, once I shift my behavior, others around me have had to as well.

One example of this is our family holidays that have been spent in a beautiful log house in the Adirondacks. This house is gorgeous, with a huge living room where everyone gathers. It also has the thinnest walls of any house I've ever been in. When I stay there with my entire family I get very little sleep, and for me the consequences of this are huge because it increases my pain level. For years I would go to this house at Christmas, end up wracked with fatigue and pain, and then feel completely isolated while everyone else was happily going about their day, and I knew I wouldn't feel better until I left. I would feel isolated because I felt that no one understood what I was going through, and I felt unsupported and not cared about. Until I decided to speak up and finally told everyone my situation and said I couldn't do it anymore. This was huge for me because I knew how much fun the others were having in this storybook cabin in the woods. I knew that if I spoke up it could put a damper on other people's fun. On the other hand, how much did I have to suffer? As much as I wished the situation would change, that magically one day I'd be able to sleep like a log with noise all around me and wake up refreshed, I knew it wasn't going to happen. Not anytime soon anyway. So, I spoke up and told people what was going on, and it turned out just fine. I ended up sleeping at a neighbor's house in blissful quiet.

You may need to let some people go. There are some people that drain you, create negativity around you, or generally do you more harm than good. These people are best kept at arm's length. And keep in mind what Confucius said, "To be wronged is nothing unless you continue to remember it." By letting those people who choose to remain stuck in negative thinking leave your life physically and emotionally, you are allowing room for more positive, courageous people that will applaud your achievements and problem solve with you about how to move toward your goals.

## Compassion

Let's go back to the very beginning of this chapter, back when we were listening to the experience of Kiril Sokoloff. When he was describing the situation he'd been in thousands of times where letting other people's ignorance put a damper on his experience do you think he was abdicating his responsibility to stand up for his own needs? Have I done that? Have you? This is not a question that I have an absolute answer to because it is one that may have a different answer at different times.

One thing to consider is that he may have been practicing pure empathy. He was able to put himself in the shoes of those around him because at one time he had been a person who had no trouble with his hearing, someone who didn't realize that background noise can eliminate any chance for a hearing impaired person to understand. He was able to place himself back there and then make a decision. What were the benefits to him of speaking up and changing everyone's experience, possibly blunting the experience of those around him to make himself more comfortable? What were the benefits of not speaking up and allowing the situation to continue unaltered, knowing he was missing out? Could he enhance his own experience by knowing that the people around him were experiencing joy? To me this is true compassion, the compassion that comes from empathy. Kiril anticipated the distress that others would feel if he spoke up and decided not to go there.

Sometimes not speaking up is the most compassionate thing to do. Sometimes being alone in your experience is okay. As I said earlier, having a chronic health issue can and will isolate you. But remember, sometimes that is okay.

Consider this:
**Isolation→Reaching Out→Understanding→Empathy→Compassion→Isolation**

Isolation, or being set apart from others, can be just as natural as the need for bonding. There is nothing wrong with being alone in your experience, only in thinking that there is something wrong with you because you are alone. Isolation can lead to compassion, one of the greatest gifts we can give and compassion can lead to isolation, one of the conditions of our existence. Having rheumatoid arthritis may isolate you, but it also brings you the incredible opportunity to strengthen bonds with those around you and arrive at a compassionate understanding of yourself and the people you share this life with.

# *Chapter Ten Worksheets*

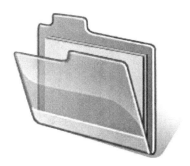

- My Bill of Rights
- Causes of Emotional Tension
- The Healing Sequence
- Steps to Effective Communication

# MY BILL OF RIGHTS

**I have the right to......**

... say "no" without feeling guilty.

....express my feelings.

....be accepted just as I am. I don't have to conform to others

    expectations about me to know that I am worthwhile.

....disagree with others and to question medical decisions regarding my

care.

....know that my arthritis does not define me.

....have a bad day occasionally.

.... talk about may pain.

.... respect myself and receive respect from others.


**Add your bill of rights here:**

....

....

....

....

....

....

....

....

# CAUSES OF EMOTIONAL TENSION

Not Feeling Cared About. Describe a situation: _____

_____

_____

_____

_____

_____

What feelings were associated with this situation? _____

_____

_____

_____

_____

_____

Not Feeling Supported. Describe a situation: _____

_____

_____

_____

_____

_____

What feelings were associated with this situation? _____

_____

_____

_____

_____

_____

Not Feeling Understood. Describe a situation: _____

_____

_____

_____

_____

_____

What feelings were associated with this situation? _____

_____

_____

_____

_____

Not Feeling Appreciated Describe a situation: _____

_____

_____

_____

_____

_____

What feelings were associated with this situation? _____

_____

_____

_____

_____

Not Feeling Respected[3] Describe a situation: _____

_____

_____

_____

_____

_____

What feelings were associated with this situation?_____

_____

_____

_____

_____

_____

[3] Adapted from *Improving Communication in Your Workplace, How to Enhance Cooperation and Minimize Conflict,* by Clarissa Russo, RN, a workbook for RN's

# THE HEALING SEQUENCE

My Trauma: _____

_____

_____

_____

My Losses: _____

_____

_____

_____

My Suffering: (what are the emotions that I feel?) _____

_____

_____

_____

My Lamenting: (How can I express how I feel to others?) _____

_____

_____

_____

Listening: (What do I need? How can I tell this[4] to others who care?) _____

_____

_____

_____

Healing!!! (List supportive people)

_____          _____

_____          _____

_____          _____

_____          _____

_____          _____

_____          _____

_____          _____

---

[4] Adapted from *Communication Skills That Heal, a practical approach to a new professionalism in medicine,* by Barry Bub MD

# STEPS TO EFFECTIVE COMMUNICATION

1. State your problem: _____
   _____
   _____
   _____

2. What are the underlying feelings that are associated with this problem? Can you identify any irrational beliefs that come from these feelings?_____
   _____
   _____
   _____

3. How have I expressed this problem in the past? _____
   _____
   _____
   _____

4. What has been the response from others? _____
   _____
   _____
   _____

5. What are my intentions now for expressing this problem to others? (To receive information, analysis, clarity, advice, understanding, reassurance, comfort, hope)
   _____
   _____
   _____
   _____

6. How can I express this problem to match my intentions? _____
   _____
   _____
   _____

*I was hiking the other day with my dog Jasper and came to a narrowing of the trail. One side was a steep hill and the other was a steep drop. I'd hiked this trail many times before and had always been careful with my step through this section. For some reason that day I took an extra look up and down and hesitated. My mind started to talk to me, telling me that no one knew where I was. If I fell it would definitely hurt and may even do damage. As I continued to imagine the worst while taking each step with trepidation, I began to slip. I slipped twice before I finally realized that my fear was controlling my body. My fear was causing my body to slip. I gingerly and gratefully made it through and shook my head.*

*Weeks later I was on the same trail with my friend Keith, deep in conversation when suddenly I stopped. I looked back and realized that I had just passed through the narrow, steep section that had caused me to falter weeks earlier.*

*We all choose what to be afraid of. Fear can save our life, but fear can cripple us as well. When fear cripples us it often does so insidiously by taking over one's mind and bringing it towards worst case scenarios. "If I walk at night I'll run into a rapist." "If I lose my job I'll lose my house." " If I leave my boyfriend I'll never find someone else." On and on until we are afraid to do anything at all. Until we stop crippling our mind, do it anyway, and find that the world doesn't come to an end.*

*As a child growing up with arthritis my worst case scenario was surgery. I knew that as long as I didn't need surgery the arthritis wasn't so bad. Then in my early twenties I was walking home from the grocery store holding a bag and I felt something pop in my right hand. Later that night I was studying with friends and realized I couldn't lift my ring finger. Ironically enough we were studying anatomy, although I really didn't need a book to tell me that not being able to lift my finger was a bad thing. The next day I went to class and told one of my occupational therapy professors what had happened. She took one look and her face fell. "Here's the number of a really good hand surgeon," she said, "Call him today."*

*Surgery. Surgeon. Words that I had always been afraid to hear. Instantly my life completely changed. By my own definition I had entered the world of someone with bad arthritis. I could no longer separate myself from other people with arthritis. Months before that fateful day I had known my hand was feeling a lot worse. It hurt to hold a utensil to eat. I had to steel myself before I lifted my wrist. It's not as if the warning signs weren't there, I had simply chosen not to look at them.*

*My fear had crippled me in two ways. It caused me to separate myself from others with "bad" arthritis and it caused me to not take positive action to help myself. But it also taught me two important lessons. When your worst fear happens life doesn't stop-the sun still shines, people keep moving through their day, and so do you. But life as you know it changes irrevocably. My perspective shifted because it had to. I knew that surgery was my worst fear because I didn't think I could accept myself as someone with arthritis. More than anything, surgery would* make the disease real and I could no longer deny it to myself and the world.

I started to let the people around me into my life with arthritis instead of just mentioning it in an offhand manner during light conversation and then expending much of my social energy trying to hide my pain. I let people become aware of the damage the arthritis in my wrist had caused. My schoolmates were occupational therapy students so they all had a scholarly interest in my predicament which made it easier for me, but as I let information leak out I found that people's acceptance of me didn't change. So, begrudgingly, I began to accept myself.

Since then my arthritis has enabled me to confront my fears time and time again, and each time my perspective has shifted. Each time I've been able to shed another layer of self-doubt and rigidity. Each time I've learned that when you break apart, you have the opportunity to rebuild a new you. Each time I've let a crippling fear leave me I feel stronger, lighter, happier, and more grateful. And I know that each time my fears allow me to know myself better.

Having arthritis means that you will face fear and each time the decision will be there for you, "Do I want to confront my fear and learn the message it contains, or do I want to be crippled by it?" To me the choice is clear.

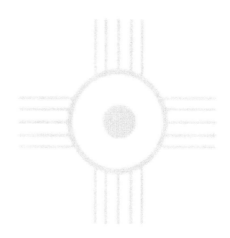

## Chapter Eleven:
A RESILIENT LIFE

*"Life is an opportunity, benefit from it.*
*Life is beauty, admire it.*
*Life is bliss, taste it.*
*Life is a dream, realize it.*
*Life is a challenge, meet it.*
*Life is a duty, complete it.*
*Life is a game, play it.*
*Life is a promise, fulfill it.*
*Life is sorrow, overcome it.*
*Life is a song, sing it.*
*Life is a struggle, accept it.*
*Life is a tragedy, confront it.*
*Life is an adventure, dare it.*
*Life is luck, make it.*
*Life is too precious, do not destroy it.*
*Life is life, fight for it."*
                    *-Mother Teresa*

Caroline Myss, Phd, a writer, teacher, and expert on energy medicine, says belief in oneself is required for healing. She also says, "There is a great power in the will to heal, and without that internal power, a disease usually has its way with the physical body." Internal power is a huge part of living a resilient life. Along with the will to heal, internal power always involves moving beyond self-limiting thoughts and toward the truths that we all hold inside.

Part of healing involves looking at what makes us feel good. We all want to feel better. Unfortunately, many people rely on the outside world to enable them to feel better about themselves. Any material object that one wants to possess is desired for the sole purpose of how that object will make them feel. We cultivate relationships that make us feel good, and most of our actions have feeling good as their ultimate purpose. Knowing this, we all have to take an honest look at ourselves and ask, "Where does my good feeling come from?"

Learning to feel good from the inside out instead of the outside in is internal power. People who feel good on the inside feel worthy and they treat themselves well. They also exude those good feelings to those around them and are able to be less judgmental and more compassionate with themselves and others. People who feel good from the inside out may be happy about owning material objects, but they don't require those objects for their happiness. People who feel good from the inside out are able to face the ever changing tides of life with equanimity because they are able to wait out the low periods, knowing that this too shall pass. People who feel good from the inside out are able to be happy alone because they take the time to know themselves and find that they are endlessly fascinating and surprising. They will laugh at this, and will laugh often at themselves and the absurdities of life. People who feel good from the inside out are able to fully relax. They are able to stop and slow down because they have no need to grasp for the next thing or person that will make them feel better. People who feel good from the inside out may have feelings of negativity such as anger, fear, anxiety, or jealousy, but they don't harbor them for long because they are able to recognize that harboring negative emotions creates more negativity and ill health. They know that these emotions hold a lesson and it's best to learn the lesson and move on.

People who feel good from the inside out have internal power because they aren't draining their energy everywhere. People who search outside themselves for clues, proof, and validation that they are worthy, who need objects or people in order to have self esteem end up draining themselves and others. You will never be able to cultivate internal power until you stop looking outside yourself and start believing in yourself. That is when the will to heal becomes the act of healing. That is the truth we have inside.

> *"Those who know others have intelligence*
> *Those who know themselves have insight*
> *Those who master others have force*
> *Those who master themselves have true power"*
>                                             *-Tao Te Jing*

Most of us need to work on feeling good from the inside out. We are an outside in society and we probably learned to be this way at a very young age. Undoing what was done to you as a child is the work of adulthood, and once you have accomplished this you will be free to unleash the gifts that you alone were meant to share with the world.

I remember when I first began this process for myself. I was in my early twenties and had just started working as an occupational therapist. I was succeeding in every conventional sense of the word. I was making a good salary and called my Dad every few months asking him how to invest all the money I was saving. I was a senior occupational therapist at my job even though I'd only been out of school for a few years. I had lots of friends, my arthritis was in control, and I had the energy to bike ride at least four times a week.

But I was constantly battling myself and my body's needs. I spent the time that I didn't feel good angry at my body for failing me. I never rested and I didn't talk about my arthritis; instead, I put on a happy face and bucked up even when I didn't want to. I chose boyfriends who had no interest in knowing the real me and lived a double life. I would go 110 miles an hour around them and then collapse by myself so my body could recuperate. I spent my recovery time feeling angry at my body. I was critical of myself and felt that I needed to do more. I was living the life I had learned to live as a kid.

I began to get sick. Weird bodily reactions made conventional doctors shake their heads and nontraditional healers put me on various detox diets. I spent time following orders from my various doctors until I became so frustrated at their ineffectiveness that I began to look inside. Not at what I was eating, or what supplement I was taking, or what medication regime I was doing, but at how I was really feeling.

For me, even knowing how I was feeling was a challenge and still is sometimes. I'd lived my entire life hiding my feelings so well that I was a master at hiding them even from myself. Occasionally, they would leak out in various ways: anorexia, overdoing it, self-recrimination. Always directed at myself, always harmful to myself. Always anger at myself.

I later found out that anger is a secondary emotion that serves to cover a more primary emotion or emotions. I didn't know at the time that my anger was covering up my more devastating feelings of despair, lack of control, and isolation. My anger came out when it did because I needed to feel something, but because I had no experience with accessing my true feelings I felt anger instead. I was lucky I felt something, though because often when I didn't allow myself to feel bad, my body did it for me. When I began to get sick at the very time, by all conventional wisdom I should have been thriving, my body was talking loud and clear.

> *"In order to heal, you must feel."*
> *-Kathryn Diane Elton*

Since that time I've learned how I really feel, and I've learned how to express my feelings in a helpful way to those around me. During this process I learned what my boundaries are and how to stick up for my needs. Just as a snake sheds its skin when it no longer needs it, I've had to shed old patterns of thinking and behaving that no longer serve me.

Instead of taking care of the needs that the arthritis creates for me in a grudging way, I am now able to pat myself on the back for being creative at solving the problems that come up. I'm able to feel grateful that I have the ability to take care of my needs. It doesn't always feel good, it isn't always easy, but it is always worth it. Acknowledging my feelings has allowed me to learn from them and allowed me to grow. It's allowed me to understand my meaning in life, my purpose for being here. And it's allowed me to begin to heal, because you can't heal yourself until you know yourself.

Caroline Myss says that your biography is your biology, Candace Pert, Phd, a neuroscientist, says that our molecules of emotion shape who we are. I say that self-knowledge and self-worth are requirements for healing. Because, without them you will never feel good from the inside out.

Resilience requires internal power because without it you won't be able to have the fortitude to take the actions that resilience requires. Resilience involves having the intention of always moving forward in a positive direction. With this intention you take action. When it comes to arthritis, many of my decisions about how to proceed aren't easy or clear cut. My hard choices can be scary, but I can still make them because I know that this is the way it's supposed to be. Some of my decisions are moving to create something, others are to accept something and I can use my self-knowledge to tell me which is the right direction to go. I always remind myself that deciding to do nothing is a decision in itself, and that keeps me focused on what I really want. I want to keep moving closer and closer to balance until the arthritis is no longer necessary. I believe that this is possible. I believe that this day will come.

Intentions are created every day whether we consciously think about them or not. The wonderful thing about making your intentions conscious is that in doing so you will be creating your life instead of just being a pawn.

The first thing that happened for me when I started to do this is that my intentions changed. In the beginning, my intentions were more like goals, coming from my ego and what I thought I should do and have. My affirmations went something like this:

- "In six months all my swelling will be gone."
- "In six months I will be working as an occupational therapist with people who have arthritis."
- "In six months I will be teaching classes in the community."
- "I ride my bike five times a week."
- "I am pain free."

My affirmations were coming from a place of fear and desperation- what I thought I had to be able to do, what I needed to do so I could accept myself. I needed to reach the Shangri La that I had created in my head. As time went on and I began to wonder why I wasn't moving forward toward my affirmations I learned a few things. I realized that affirmations have to come from a deep place inside. The place that knows my purpose for being here, instead of my ego which tries to force the ideas of "should," and, "need to," that I learned as a child. I realized that it's within my rights as a human who wants to thrive to ask to not be in pain, ask to be free from the arthritis, but it's also my duty to let go, surrender my will, and know that there is a divine timing to all things. Deepak Chopra talks about the "Law of Intention and Desire" in his book, *The Seven Spiritual Laws of Success*, and he says, "Intention is the real power behind desire. Intent alone is very powerful, because intent alone is desire without attachment to the outcome. Intention combined with detachment leads to life centered, present moment awareness. And when action is performed in present moment awareness, it is most effective. Your intent is for the future, but your intent for the future will manifest, because the future is created in the present. You must accept the present as is. Accept the present and intend the future. The future is something you can create through detached intention, but you should never struggle against the present."

As time went on my intentions shifted from being forceful and rigid, and became more gentle and uplifting. Thoughts like:
- "I take positive steps every day to help my body feel better."

- "I find new ways to create sound sleep for myself."
- "I have a job I love that uses my skills and still leaves me the energy to live a balanced life."
- "I move closer everyday towards balance in my body until the arthritis is no longer necessary."

Having intentions that you hold close is like planting seeds. Creating your seeds involves letting go of your ego and beginning to reach deeper inside. Paying attention to them every day will allow them to grow. Shouting loudly at them won't make them sprout any faster. You nurture your seeds of intention every day through belief, positive action, and detachment, or letting go of the outcome. As the Buddha said, "The secret of health for both the mind and body is not to mourn for the past, not to worry about the future, not to anticipate troubles, but to live in the present wisely and earnestly."

The source for resiliency comes from your spirit. The ephemeral concept that we all struggle to define. There are as many descriptions of spirit as there are religions, colors of skin, or cultures. Spirit is older than civilization itself.

To me, my spirit is the deep wisdom that lies beneath the chaos of my mind. My spirit is there for me like a wise elder that gently guides me toward knowing if I let him. I can live in this world without acknowledging my spirit, but I know that in order to live well I need to talk to my spirit often enough so I don't veer too far off course. The spirit never gets weary because it draws from an eternal well of love. My spirit will never turn its back on me. My spirit is where I find my compassion for myself, which is the greatest healer of all. From my spirit I forgive myself, I hold onto my belief in myself, and I know. I know that curing isn't a requirement for healing, but healing is a requirement for curing. And I know that in order to heal my body, I need to heal my mind.

For much of my life I existed in survival mode. Resting was a foreign concept to me throughout my childhood as I struggled to keep up. When I wasn't struggling to keep up I was working hard to put on the happy face that I knew I needed to have. Because I didn't express any emotions other than, "I'm good, I'm fine," I became numb.

Numbness is a good survival technique. It stops you from getting hurt and enables you to push forward. Numbness gives you the false impression that you can get through on your own. However, being numb makes for bad decision-making. The decisions I made when I was still numb and continuing to act out my childhood scenario kept me in survival mode, kept me from having comfort as a part of my life. During this time I did "cure" the arthritis for a time, but I didn't stay there because I kept pushing myself, pushing harder at myself until the "cure" had dissolved. I was nowhere close to being healed.

What I know now with the 20/20 vision that hindsight and growth provides is that although survival mode serves a purpose by keeping us alive through difficult times, in order to thrive you must shift out of it. Sometimes life pounds us with stress, divorce, death, financial woes, illness, and we have to do what we can do to get through the day. The problem is that many of us continue to stay in survival mode because we've been accustomed to being there and we're not in touch with the inner wisdom of our spirit. There is no way you can heal your body if you are in survival mode. When you are in survival mode you are dangerously close to falling down the rabbit hole into raging disease. If you are living in survival mode you need to get out of it as soon as you can.

The first thing to do is to forgive yourself for being there in the first place and then move on. The second thing to do is to use your strengths to help you climb back into comfort and avoid turning them into weaknesses. Two strengths I have are my internal fortitude and strong will. When I was in survival mode I used these qualities to push myself. Now I use them to help myself be as healthy and comfortable as I can every day. When I was in survival mode I used my will to achieve what I considered to be my perfect life, remission. Once I was in remission I would give myself everything I wanted, I would become this person that finally was deserving. Now I know that this fantasy of the Shangri La I would live in only when I got rid of the arthritis prevented me from creating the perfect life with what I already had in front of my face.

The saying, "It takes a village to raise a child," could apply to living resiliently with rheumatoid arthritis. You will have a hard time doing this on your own. And it will be impossible to stay out of survival mode for very long if you don't have help. Learning to reach out and accept help was, and continues to be, a huge lesson for me. Asking for help makes the fact that I can't do something a reality. It reminds me that I have less energy reserves and physical strength than I otherwise would have had rheumatoid arthritis not decided to settle in my joints. However, the consequences of not receiving help can be huge. Throughout the years I let my stubbornness override my good sense I ended up increasing the stress on my joints and probably did some irreparable damage.

There is one day that has become forever ingrained into my memories as an "aha" moment. My first job was working in a for-profit rehabilitation hospital and it was very fast paced and unforgiving. The therapists would see patients every half an hour and I ended up racing down the hallways to keep up. We would all spend our lunch hour doing paperwork because we didn't have a moment to spare during the day. Not surprisingly, the hospital went through therapists like baseball players go through bats.

One day I was treating a patient that had severe rheumatoid arthritis. She was in her sixties and had raised four children. Like everyone I've ever met who's had this disease for any length of time she was a trooper, didn't complain and did anything I asked. I was adapting a pen so she could hold it to write, when she said something out of the blue. "I shouldn't have washed so many diapers by hand. I would wring them tightly until they didn't drip and I hurt my hands." The look on her face was the epitome of regret and sadness. It stopped me in my tracks because during that time in my life I was pushing the arthritis to the background, hiding its troublesome nature from myself and everyone around me. I had chosen a job that no sane person would have wanted unless they were desperate, a job that was causing even the most physically hardy of folks to end up hurting their backs, and deep down inside, below the layer of self-denial I knew that I was making a big mistake. I was trying to do the right thing, be successful, be "normal," and was only succeeding in creating regrets for myself. I wish I could say that I got the message right then and there and quit my job immediately, but I didn't. What I can say is that I know that right now, living my life in a resilient manner, I'm not creating more regrets. The day I stopped creating regrets was the day that I stopped needing to prove my self-worth and started to live as though I was already worthy.

Part of what this looks like is having a wide circle of support so that you don't have to hurt yourself in any way. You already hurt enough. Service to others is one duty that comes with being human and anytime you give to another it is clear that the rewards you get in return are greater than any sacrifice you had to make. If we live a life that includes service to others we will begin to see our circle of support widen. And we won't feel so bad about asking for the help we need.

The village that it takes to live well with rheumatoid arthritis includes different things for different people but will always include methods to improve your physical comfort level, people to support you emotionally, and people who can help you physically. Without these things you will be too close to walking the line, the line that crossing will put you back into survival mode and too close to ill-health.

This disease we call rheumatoid arthritis, as I said in the first sentence in this book, isn't for sissies. It has driven grown men to drink, socialites to turn into recluses, has caused people to suffer in innumerable ways, and most heartbreaking of all, can strip away your belief. Letting go of the doubt that will inevitably course through our thoughts as we wake up day after day with swollen joints, even as we are doing every possible thing we know of to help the arthritis to subside, could probably humble even the Buddha himself. Resiliency comes from within.

The belief that allows you to thrive is believe in yourself, believe that no matter what your present circumstance is now, you are always in the process of changing and you can change for the better just as easily as you can change for the worse. People who thrive accept the unpredictability of life and use it to create opportunity. People who thrive learn to stop struggling against their reality and adapt to whatever circumstance life brings them. Belief in yourself allows you to feel good about your choices. When it comes to rheumatoid arthritis there are no clear cut answers. The important thing to remember is that feeling good about what you are doing is often more important than what you are actually doing. This means that allowing yourself to get talked into a treatment for arthritis that you don't feel good about is a bad idea. Believe in yourself because when it comes to your body you are the only real expert.

Above all, a resilient life with arthritis means doing your best, each day. As the author of *The Four Agreements*, Don Miguel Ruiz, says, your best will be different every day, but as long as you do your best with what you have, you will avoid regrets and self judgment. I do my best every day because I know that my life is a precious gift and I want to enjoy it as much as I can. I know that you're never given anything you can't handle, so I know I can handle this day. I know that doing my best is often different from what I want it to be, but that's okay. I know that if I do my best every day I am fulfilling my purpose for being here. And I know this gift that I call my life is a miracle created just for me.

# *Chapter Eleven Worksheet*

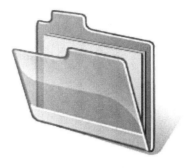

- My Resilient Life

# MY RESILIENT LIFE

What are my greatest fears about the arthritis? How have they crippled me? How can I face them and let them go? _____

_____

_____

_____

_____

What beliefs do I still hold from my childhood about myself and the world that are keeping from feeling good on the inside? What patterns of thinking no longer serve me? _____

_____

_____

_____

_____

How can I feel good from the inside out? _____

_____

_____

_____

_____

What is my purpose for being here, the meaning of my life? What gifts do I bring to the world and how can I use them to be of service?_____

_____

_____

_____

_____

What affirmations or intentions can I use to move my life forward in a positive direction?

_____

_____

_____

_____

Can I accept the present and intend the future? _____

_____

_____

_____

_____

How can I get in touch with my spirit? _____

_____

_____

_____

_____

Am I in survival mode? If so, how can I forgive myself? What strengths will I use to get myself
out of it? _____

_____

_____

_____

_____

Who is in my village? (Friends, family, massage therapists, doctors, osteopaths, healers, etc.)

_____

_____

_____

_____

_____

_____

_____

_____

## MY RESILIENT LIFE

Use this space to write, draw, or anything else you can think of to show yourself your resilient life.

# Ordering Information:

**To order copies of this book, please visit the following website:**
www.KatElton.com

# Bibliography

[1] Fishman, Scott, and Lisa Berger. *The War on Pain.* New York; HarperCollins Publishers, 2000.

[2] Melzack, Ronald, and Patrick Wall.(1965) Pain Mechanisms, a New Theory.*Science,*150:171-179.

[3] Caudill, Margaret A. *Managing Pain Before It Manages You.* New York: The Guilford Press. 1995.

[4] Armstrong, Lance, and Sally Jenkins. *Every Second Counts.* New York; Broadway Publishers, 2004.

[5] Cutler, Howard C., and the Dalai Lama. *The Art of Happiness, a Handbook for Living.* New York; Penguin Putnam Inc., 1998.

[6] Simon, L., Lipman, A., Jacox, A., Claudill- Slosberg, M., Gill, L., Keith, F., Kerr, K., Minor, M., Sherry, D., Vallerand, A., and Vasudevan, S. *Guideline for the Management of Arthritis Pain in Osteoarthritis, Rheumatoid Arthritis, and Juvenile Chronic Arthritis, $2^{nd}$ Edition.* Glenview, Ill; American Pain Society, 2002.

[7] Goldfarb, Silvia, and Roberta W. Waddell. *Relieving Pain Naturally.* Garden City Park, NY; Square One Publishers, 2005.

[8] Goldfarb, Silvia, and Roberta W. Waddell. *Relieving Pain Naturally.* Garden City Park, NY; Square One Publishers, 2005.

[9] Watson, Ann(2007, June). *Cognitive Restructuring: Changing Your Mind to Change Your Mood.*Presented atClinical Training in Mind/Body Medicine, Boston, Massachusetts,pps. 137-143.

[10] University of Washington, *Acute Inflammation* (Online). Available:http://courses.washington.edu/conj/inflammationacuteinflam.htm (accessed 12 March 2008)

[11] The John Hopkins Arthritis Center, *Rheumatoid Arthritis Pathophysiology* (Online). Available:http://www.hopkins-arthritis.org/arthritis-info/rheumatoid-arthritis/rheum_clin_path.html (accessed 12 Marc 2008)

[12] Humber,D.(1996)*Introduction to Immunology,* (Online),

Available:http://homepages.uel.ac.uk/d.p.humber/immunol.htm
(accessed 12 March 2008)

[13]Wikipedia.adapted from *History of Immunology,*(2008*)Timeline of Immunology.*(Online),
Available:http://en.wikipedia.org/wiki/History_of_immunology(accessed 12 March 2008)

[14] Sompayrac, L.,*How the Immune System Works, 2nd Edition.* New York: Blackwell Publishing, 2003

[15] Nossal, G.J.V.,*Life, Death, and the Immune System.* Sept. 1993; Scientific American Magazine A Special Issue, p 79.

[16] Sompayrac, L.,*How the Immune System Works, 2nd Edition.* New York: Blackwell Publishing, 2003.

[17] Balandraud, N., et al. Epstein Barr Virus Load in the Peripheral Blood of Patients with Rheumatoid Arthritis: Accurate quantification using real-time polymerase chain reactions,*Arthritis and Rheumatism,* 5(2003):1223-8.

[18] Edwards, J., (1998). *Rheumatoid Arthritis and Autoimmunity: A new Approach to their cause & how long term cure might be achieved.* (Online), Available: http://www.ucl.ac.uk/-regfjxe/Arthritis.htm (accessed 9 November 2006)

[19] Behrens, F., Himsel, A., Rehart, S., Stanczyk, J., Beutel, B., Zimmermann, S. Y, Koehl, U., Moller, B., Gay, S., Kaltwasser, J. P, Pfeilschifter, J. M, Radeke, H. H (2007). Imbalance in distribution of functional autologous regulatory T cells in rheumatoid arthritis. *Ann Rheum Dis* 66: 1151-1156

[20] Mann, D.L.(2008, January).Rheumatoid Arthritis and Food Allergies. January. 2008;*Arthritis Today Magazine.*

[21] Lewey, Dr. Scot. "How the Immune System Works & Fails Resulting in Autoimmune Disease, Leaky Gut, And Food Allergies."15 Jul. 2007. *EzineArticles.com.* 16 May.

[22] Eskandari,, F., Webster, J., and Sternberg, E. (2003). Neural Immune Pathways and their Coneecton to Rheumatoid Arthritis. *Arthritis Research and Therapy* 5: 251-265.

[23] Aboutarthritiscom. *The Facts of Corticosteroids.* (Online). Available:http://www.arthritis-about.com (accessed 20 March 2008).

[24] Chan, E., and Cronstein, B. (2002). Molecular Action of Methotrexate in Inflammatory Diseases. *Arthritis Research and Therapy* 4:266-273.

[25] Aboutarthritis.com. *Treatments.* (Online). Available:http://www.arthrtis-about.com (accessed 20 March 2008),

[26] John Hopkins Arthritis Center.*Rheumatoid Arthritis Treatment.* (Online). Available: http://www.hopkins-arthritis.org/arthritis-info/rheumatoid-arthritis/rheum-treat.html

[27] Sompayrac, L.,*How the Immune System Works, 2nd Edition.* New York: Blackwell Publishing, 2003.

[28] Bathon, J.,(2007)*Rheumatoid Arthritis Pathophysiology.*(Online), Available:http://www.hopkins_arthritis-som.jhmi.edu/rheumatoid/rheum_clin_path.html (accessed 14 March 2008)

[29] Sompayrac, L.,*How the Immune System Works, 2nd Edition.* New York: Blackwell Publishing, 2003.

[31] Nugent, Steve. *How to Survive on a Toxic Planet, 2nd Edition.* The Alethia Corporation, 2004.

[32] Soil Association. *Myth and Reality, Organic vs. Non-Organic: The Facts.* (Online), Available:http://www.farmingsolutions.org. (accessed 15 May 2008).

[33] U.S. Food and Drug Administration.*Nutritional Info Available for Raw Fruits, Vegetables, Fish.* (Online), Available: http://www.fda.gov/fdac/special/foodlabel/raw/html. (accessed 1 June 2008).

[34] That's Fit. *Top Five VegesEaten By American.*(Online), Available: http://www.thatsfit.com/2008/05/24/top-five-veges-eaten-by-americans (accessed 30 May 2008)

[35] Weil, Andrew. *Healthy Aging, A Lifelong Guide To Your Physical and Spiritual Well-Being.* New York, N.Y.: Alfred Knopf, 2005.

[36] Health Castle. *Trans fats 101.* (Online), Available: http://www.healthcastle.com/trans.shtml (accessed 2 June 2008).

[37] Ban Trans Fats. *About Trans Fat.* (Online), Available: http://www.bantransfats/abouttransfat.html (accessed 2 June 2008).

[38] Reinagel, Monica, with Julius Torelli, M.D. *The Inflammation free Diet Plan.* New York, N.Y.: McGraw-Hill, 2006. Pgs. 3-4.

[39] Reinagel, Monica, with Julius Torelli, M.D. *The Inflammation free Diet Plan.* New York, N.Y. : McGraw-Hill, 2006.

[40] Reinagel, Monica, with Julius Torelli, M.D. *The Inflammation free Diet Plan.* New York, N.Y.: McGraw-Hill, 2006.

[41] University of Maryland. *Functional Food Research Wins Yu Young*

*scientist Award.* (Online), Available:
http://www.newsdesk.umd.edu/scitech/release.cfm?ArticleID=1353.
(accessed 4 June 2008).

[42] Jensen, Gordon, MD PhD. *Inflammation as the Key Interface of the Medical and Nutritional Universes: A provocative Examination of the Future of Medicine and Nutrition.* (Online), Available:
http://pen.sagepub.com/cgi/content/full/30/5/453#TBL5. (accessed 5 June 2008).

[43] Srivastava,K, and T. Mustafa.*Ginger in Rheumatism and Musculoskeletal Disorders.* (Online), Available:
http://www.ncbi.nlm.nih.gov/pubmed

[44] Weil, Andrew. *Healthy Aging, A Lifelong Guide To Your Physical and Spiritual Well-Being.* New York, N.Y.: Alfred Knopf, 2005. Pgs 33, 168-9.

[45] Regenerative Nutrition. *Cayenne Pepper.* (Online), Available:
http://www.regenerativenutrition.com/content.asp?id=133 (accessed 12 June 2008).

[46] Balch, Phyliss C.N.C., and James Balch, M.D. *Prescription for Dietary Wellness.* Garden City Park, N.Y.: Avery Publishing, 1992,1998.

[47] Pitchford, Paul. *Healing With Whole Foods.* Berkeley, California.: North Atlantic Books, 1993.

[48] Eustice, Carol and Richard. *Vitamin C and Arthritis: Research Reveals Effect of Vitamin C on Joint.* (Online), Available:
http://about.arthritis.com/od/preventionandriskfactors/a/vitaminchtm.
(accessed 12 June 2008).

[49] Adam, O. et al. Anti-inflammatory Effects of a Low Arachidonic acid Diet and Fish Oil in Patients with Rheumatoid Arthritis,*Rheumatology International* 23 (2003): 27-36.

[50] Kavanagh,R. et al. The Effects of Elemental Diet and Subsequent Food Reintroduction on Rheumatoid Arthritis, *Rheumatology* 34 (1995): 270-273.

[51] Hafstrom, B et al. A vegan diet free of gluten improves the signs and symptoms of rheumatoid arthritis:The effects on arthritis correlate with the reduction in antibodies to food antigens, *Rheumatology* 40 (2001): 1175-79.

[52] Miller, C. Exercise is part of a Healthy Lifestyle for Rheumatoid Arthritis (Online), Available:http://www.healthcentral.com/rheumatoid-arthritis/c/38/19936/part/?ic=4027.(accessed 30 June 2008)

[53] Khalsa,S.B.(2007, June).*Managing Sleep disorders with Mind / Body*

*Medicine.*Presented atClinical Training in Mind/Body Medicine, Boston, Massachusetts,p. 390.

[54] Khalsa,S.B.(2007, June).*Managing Sleep disorders with Mind / Body Medicine.*Presented atClinical Training in Mind/Body Medicine, Boston, Massachusetts,p. 389.

[55] Dement, William C. *The Promise of Sleep, A Pioneer in Sleep Medicine Explores the Vital Connection Between Health, Happiness, and a Good Night's Sleep.* New York, N.Y.: Dell Publishing, 1999.pgs. 18-23.

[56]Khalsa,S.B.(2007, June).*Managing Sleep disorders with Mind / Body Medicine.*Presented atClinical Training in Mind/Body Medicine, Boston, Massachusetts, pgs. 390-91.

[57] Hauri, Peter, and Linde, Shirley. *No More Sleepless Nights.* New York, N.Y.: John Wiley and Sons, 1990, 1996.pgs. 23-4.

[58] Lasley, F. A Review of Sleep in Selected Immune and Autoimmune Disorders. *Holistic Nurse Practitioner* 17 (2003): 65-80.

[59] Hauri, Peter, and Linde, Shirley. *No More Sleepless Nights.* New York, N.Y.: John Wiley and Sons, 1990, 1996. p. 18.

[60] Hauri, Peter, Jarman, Murray, and Shirley Linde. *No More Sleepless Nights Workbook, Tracking your Progress Toward a Great Night's Sleep.* New York, N.Y.: John Wiley and Sons, 2001.p. 54.

[61] Jacobs, Gregg. *Say Goodnight to Insomnia, The 6-Week Solution, A Drug Free Program Developed at Harvard Medical School.* New York, N.Y.: Owl Books, 1998. p.81.

[62] Jacobs, Gregg. *Say Goodnight to Insomnia, The 6-Week Solution, A Drug Free Program Developed at Harvard Medical School.* New York, N.Y.: Owl Books, 1998.p. 124.

[63] Balch, James F., and Phyliss A Balch. *Prescription for Nutritional Healing.* Garden City Park, N.Y.:Avery Publishing Group Inc., 1990.p. 222.

[64]Jacobs, Gregg. *Say Goodnight to Insomnia, The 6-Week Solution, A Drug Free Program Developed at Harvard Medical School.* New York, N.Y.: Owl Books, 1998.p. 108.

[65] Jacobs, Gregg. *Say Goodnight to Insomnia, The 6-Week Solution, A Drug Free Program Developed at Harvard Medical School.* New York, N.Y.: Owl Books, 1998.pgs 113-114.

[66] Dement, William C. *The Promise of Sleep, A Pioneer in Sleep Medicine Explores the Vital Connection Between Health, Happiness, and a Good Night's Sleep.* New York, N.Y.: Dell Publishing, 1999.p. 373.

[67] Jacobs, Gregg. *Say Goodnight to Insomnia, The 6-Week Solution, A Drug*

*Free Program Developed at Harvard Medical School.* New York, N.Y.: Owl Books, 1998.p. 95.

[68] Khalsa,S.B.(2007, June).*Managing Sleep disorders with Mind / Body Medicine.*Presented atClinical Training in Mind/Body Medicine, Boston, Massachusetts. p. 405.

[69] Hauri, Peter, and Linde, Shirley. *No More Sleepless Nights.* New York, N.Y.: John Wiley and Sons, 1990, 1996.p. 80.

[70] Dement, William C. *The Promise of Sleep, A Pioneer in Sleep Medicine Explores the Vital Connection Between Health, Happiness, and a Good Night's Sleep.* New York, N.Y.: Dell Publishing, 1999.p. 169.

[71] Bub, Barry. *Communication Skills that Heal, a practical approach to a new professionalism in medicine.* Oxon: Radcliffe Publishing, 2006 (p.102)

[72] Benson, Herbert, and Eileen M. Stuart. *The Wellness Workbook, The Comprehensive Guide To Maintaining Health and Treating Stress Related Illness.* New York, N.Y.: Simon & Schuster (1992).

9 780615 289236